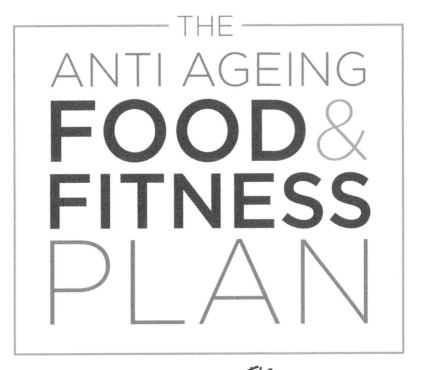

THE
ANTI AGEING
FOOD &
FITNESS
PLAN

BY RICK HAY *The* **SuperFoodist**

Contributors

Fitness Plan Creator
Ian Chapman

Graphic Design
Robbie Mason

Recipe and Design Advisors
Daniela Fischer
Bryan James
Vicky Hadley

Photography
Cover Photo by Andrew Cotterill

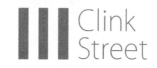

Published by Clink Street Publishing 2016
Copyright © 2016
First edition.

ISBN: 978-1-910782-57-6
E-Book: 978-1-910782-58-3

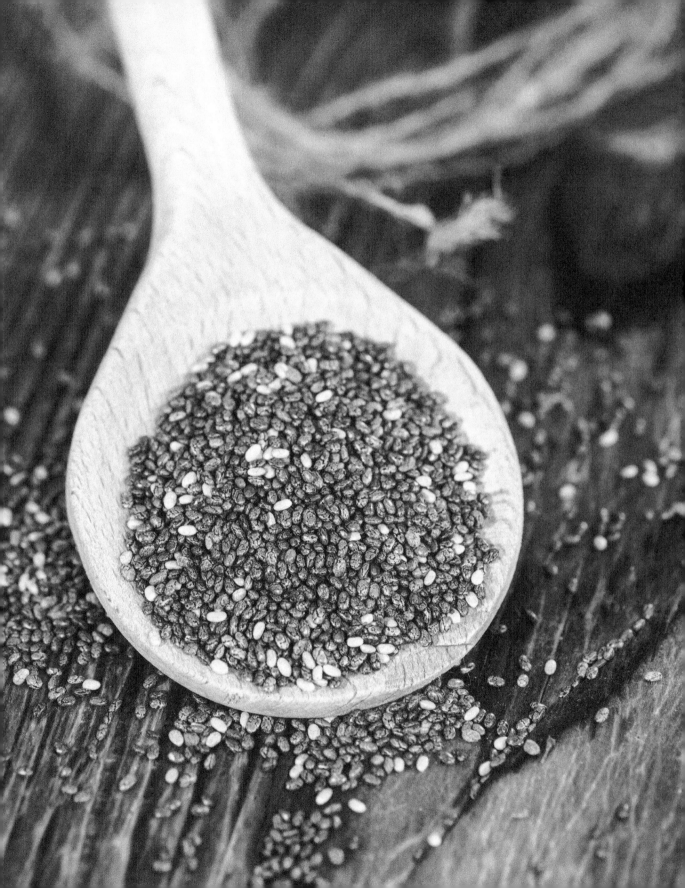

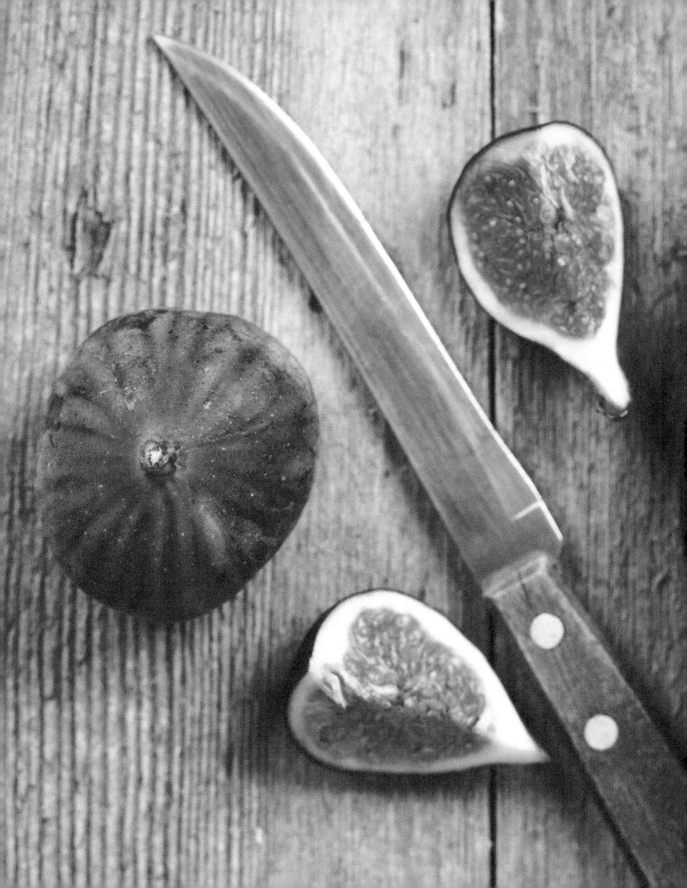

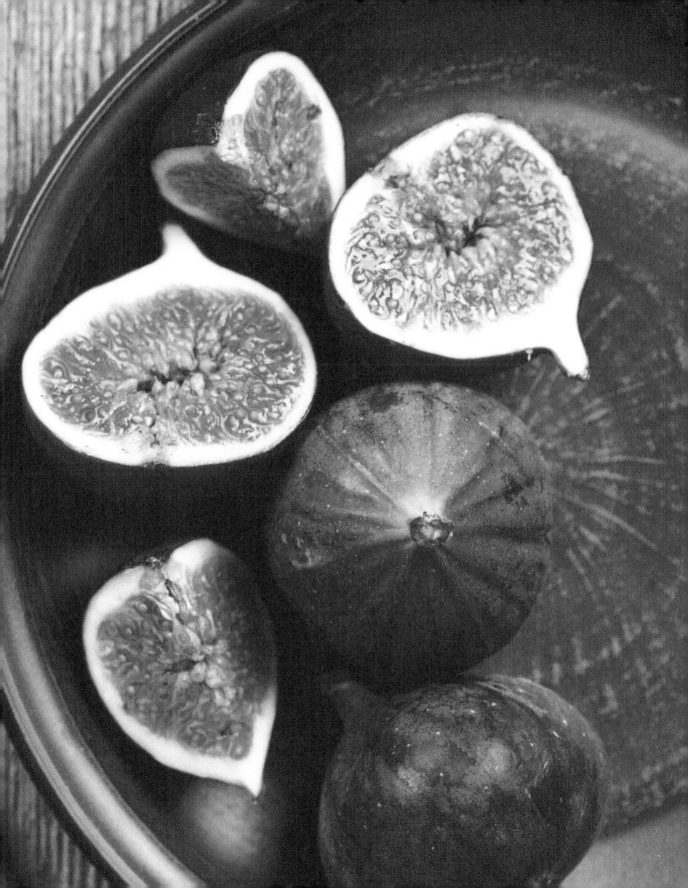

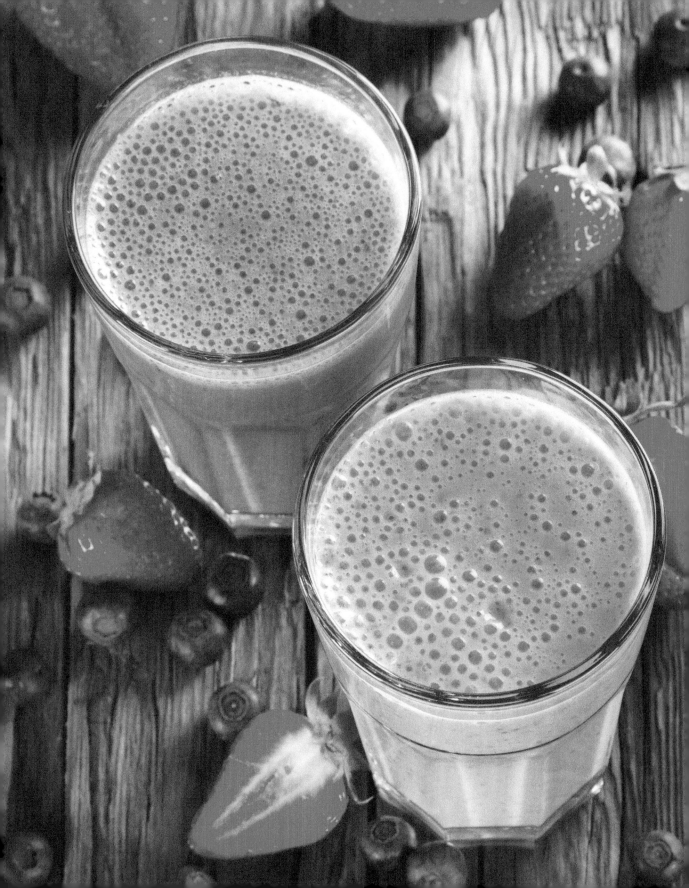

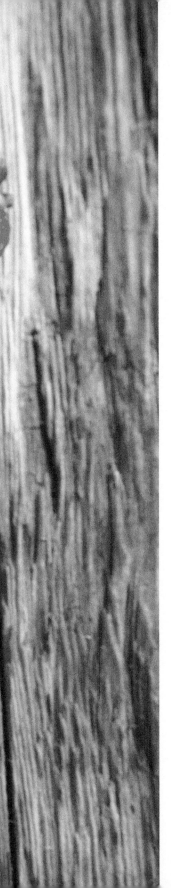

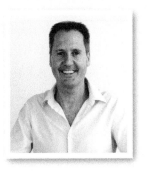

Rick Hay The Super Foodist – Dip Nutrition, Dip Botanical Medicine, Dip Iridology, Dip Teaching

Rick is an anti ageing and fitness nutritionist with many years clinical experience in nutrition, naturopathy, botanical medicine and iridology.

His specialisms include obesity treatment, weight management, anti-ageing nutraceuticals, beauty from within supplements and natural sports medicine options.

Rick lectures in Weight Management and Detox at The College of Naturopathic Medicine in London and is the Resident Health and Fitness Expert for Ideal World TV and Body In Balance.
He is also a Nutritional Ambassador for Sunwarrior, Synergy Natural and Yoogaia in the UK.

He writes a regular Natural Health and Fitness Blog for Healthista, is the Nutritional Supplement Formulator for Fushi and Co-Formulator of Believe Beauty Breakfast Cereal.

He has vast experience in nutraceutical formulation and has just released his new Superfood range - Go Figa, Go Boost and Go Green.

Rick is the author of the *Anti-Ageing Food and Fitness Plan, Nutritional Blast* and is the creator of the libido boosting 'The Little Red Dress Diet'.
He has also released three Vibrapower Fitness DVD's in conjunction with Ideal World TV.

Sarah Parish

British Film, TV and Theatre Actor

With my hectic schedule I was finding it increasingly more difficult to stay in shape.
I was looking for something that would provide results that were achievable and sustainable - I wanted to get in shape the smart way.

When I met Rick and looked into the science behind both the healthy eating and fitness components of the plan I was really impressed.
Fad diets or complicated exercise regimes are definitely not what I need.

The nutritional philosophy really resonates with me - The Anti Ageing Food & Fitness Plan delivers nutrient density, cellular health and anti ageing benefits with no calorie counting!
I'm even an expert on telomeres now!

I love that I'm looking and feeling better - these 12 weeks could see you healthily drop a dress size, tone up and turn back the clock!

Sarah Parish

P.S. The recipes are delicious and easy to prepare and the fitness sections are fast and effective!

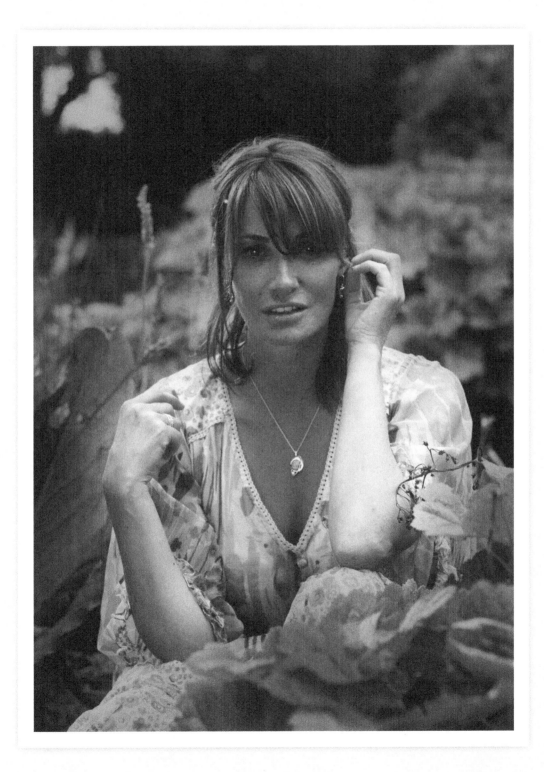

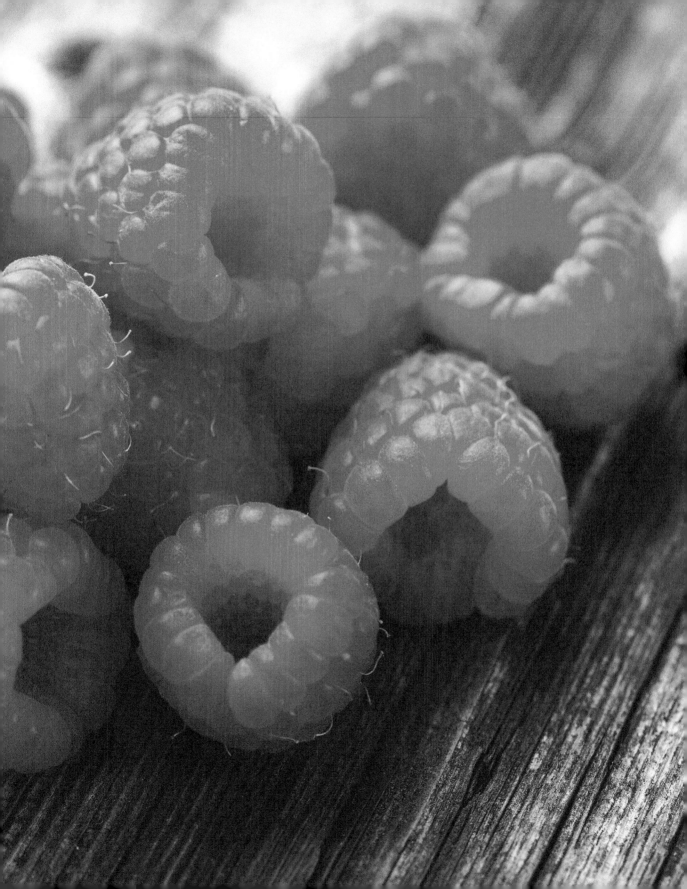

CONTENTS

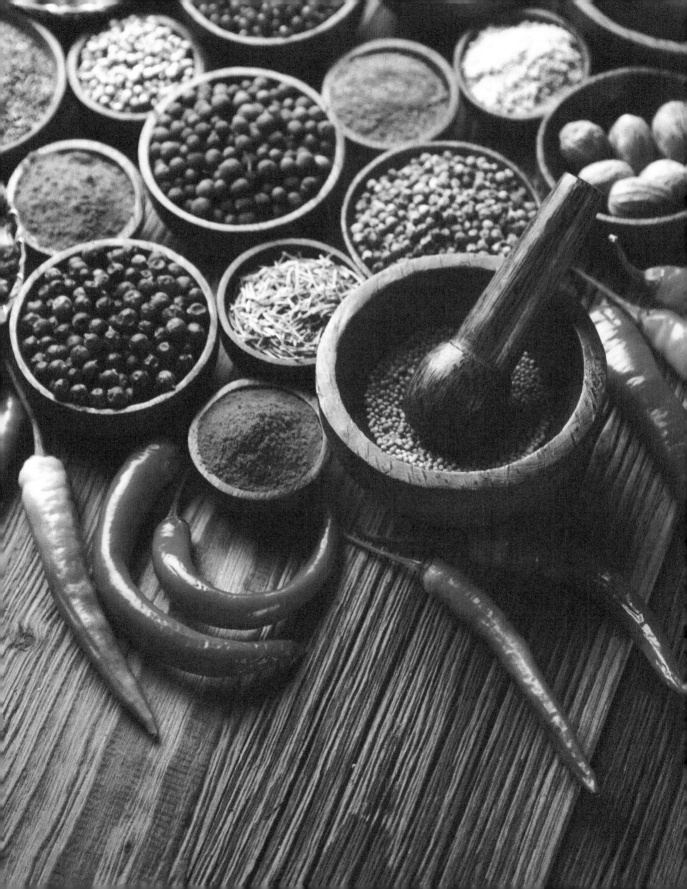

INTRODUCTION

The Anti Ageing Food and Fitness Plan has been designed to achieve the best anti ageing, fitness and weight loss outcomes over a **12 week period.**

The plan is easy to follow and targets ageing and fitness at a cellular level using nutrient dense meals, snacks, supplements and high intensity interval training.

The selected foods, herbs and spices promote fat metabolism and improve digestive function whilst helping to control cravings and improve satiety.

The meals and snacks provide low glycaemic load nutrient density to keep blood sugar levels steady and to boost both immunity and energy production.
The first four weeks have been designed to tune your body up. The Tune Up phase is followed by Rev Up, which is the second four weeks, with the last four week Tone Up section being all about weight management and toning.

Plant Based Protein such as Sunwarrior is recommended throughout the plan to increase the protein content of the smoothies - this will keep you fuller for longer and also help to keep cravings at bay.

You can also use any of the Superfood Nutraceuticals from my Go range - Go Figa, Go Boost or Go Green to increase the nutrient levels of the juices or smoothies.

In addition I have included additional information on some recommended Nutraceuticals and Skin Care products to enhance results.

What's it all about?

Eating a diet that is predominantly made up of nutrient dense plant based protein has been shown to increase life expectancy whilst lowering the incidence of many of today's common disease states such as cardiovascular problems, diabetes and obesity related illnesses.

At a cellular level the nutrient dense meal and snack options that are included in this plan have been chosen to optimise cellular function and to provide your body with all of the vitamins, minerals, electrolytes, antioxidants and phytonutrients that are required in order to achieve optimal health.

Providing the body with the right fuel optimises the trillions of biochemical reactions that take place every minute inside your body. Some of these nutrients are being shown to help increase cellular life and to lengthen and protect telomeres - which in turn leads to a longer life span.

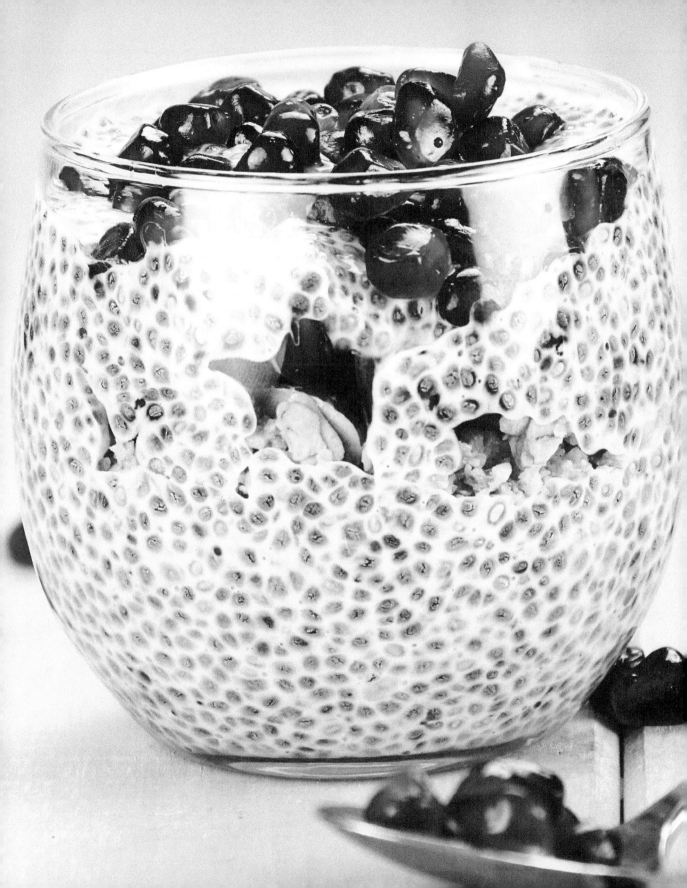

The food choices help with alkalisation and detoxification and will also help you to achieve correct digestive function - if your body is not eliminating correctly, the resulting toxic build up can speed up the ageing process and hamper any weight management campaign.

Spices are included in the plan as they are thermogenic and can have a positive effect on feelings of satiety and fat oxidisation. They also help to boost the immune system and have strong anti-inflammatory properties.

The consumption of these spices increases thermogenesis throughout the day and when combined with the intermittent fasting element of the plan may help to extend lifespan.

The first four weeks are all about a tune up and include low GL recipes to promote healthy digestive, immune, lymphatic and nervous system function. The recommended exercises will enhance this initial tune up period.

The healthy protein plant based smoothies are recommended in Weeks 5 to 8 in order to kick start your metabolism and to set your body up for fat loss.

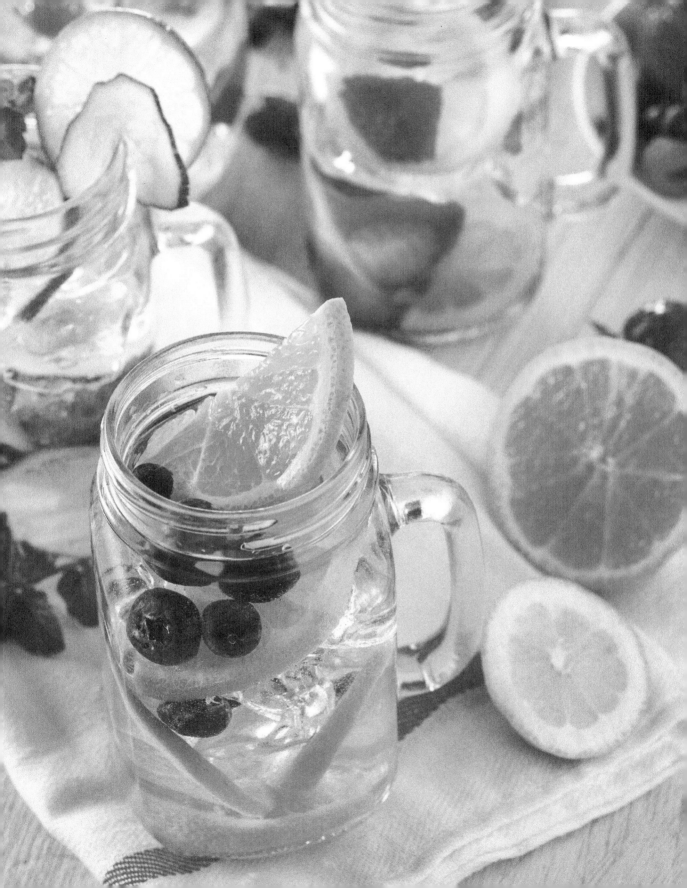

Calorie restriction is included in Weeks 9 to 12 as the research surrounding the restriction of calories is revealing that this 5/2 method of healthy eating can promote both weight loss and longevity.

The plan is not about counting calories as such but is focused on healthy food options that will deliver improved health outcomes whilst maintaining a healthy weight.

HIIT (High Intensity Interval Training) also reduces telomere shortening which helps to slow down the ageing process.

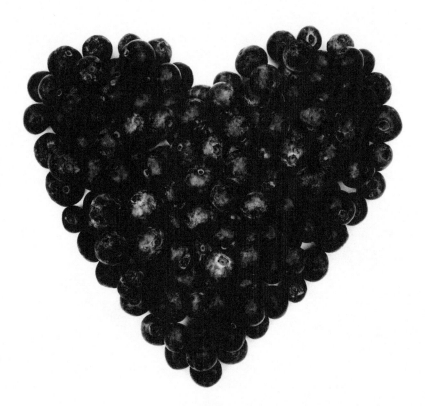

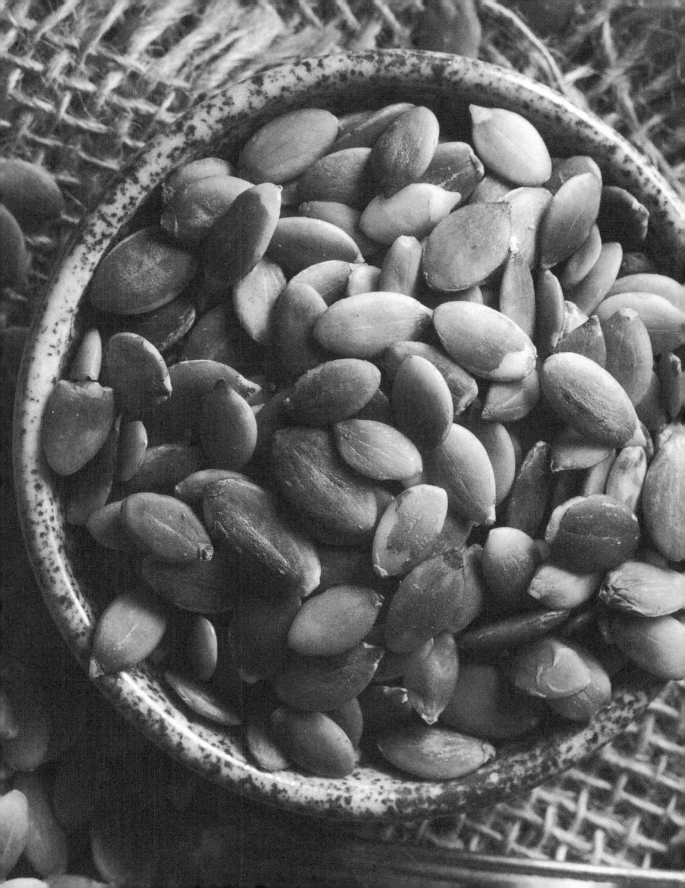

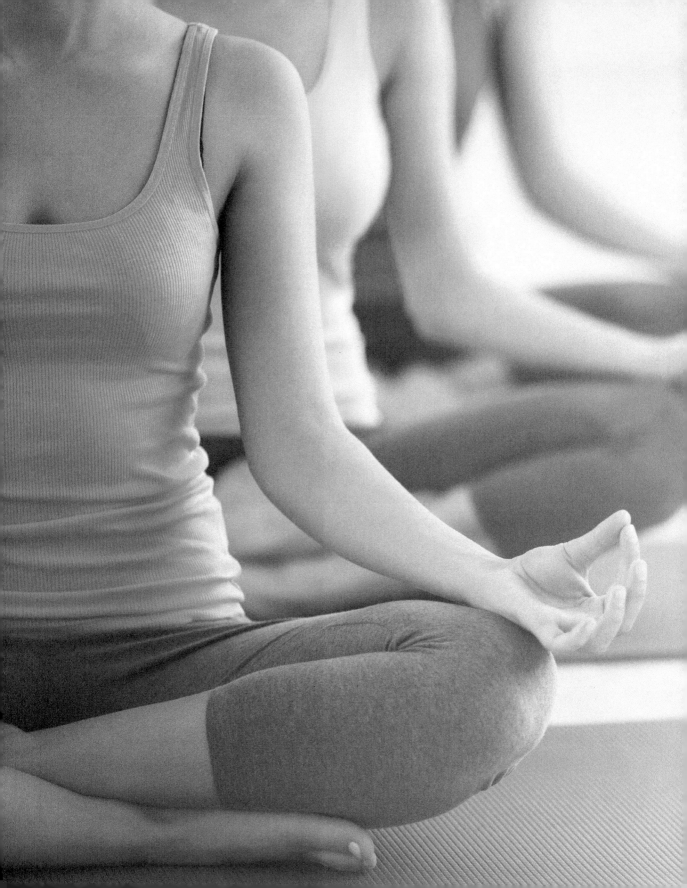

Fitness Instructions

Exercise should form an integral part of any diet plan as movement is one of the best ways to reverse or slow down the ageing process.
Research shows that even short bursts of exercise can help prevent and protect against an array of modern health issues.

Aim to implement movement and exercise into your daily routine and set approximately 3-4 times a week to do the specific exercise routines outlined in the Fitness Sections of your Anti Ageing Food and Fitness Plan.

The Cardio Circuit Challenges are based on the principle of HIIT - High Intensity Interval Training or Burst Training.
HIIT is where intervals of low to moderate intensity training is alternated with short bursts of high intensity intervals.

This style of exercise creates a super charged cardio routine which enables you to burn fat at a faster rate and in less time.
High Intensity Interval Training helps to speed up your metabolism and to burn more calories throughout the day - even after you finish exercising.

These exercises utilise your own body weight but if you wish to use some hand weights this will increase the resistance.

If you are a **Beginner** do each circuit once or twice giving you a total of **5-10 minutes** of HIIT/Cardio.

If you are **Intermediate** do each circuit two or three times giving you a total of **10-15 minutes** of HIIT/Cardio.

If you are **Advanced** do each circuit three or four times giving you a total of **15-20 minutes** of HIIT/Cardio.

HIIT Weeks 1-4
Do each exercise in the circuit for 20 seconds intensely and then slowly for 40 seconds.
Each individual exercise within the circuit should be done for 1 minute.

HIIT Week 5-8
Do each exercise in the circuit for 30 seconds intensely and then slowly for 30 seconds.
Each individual exercise within the circuit should be done for 1 minute.

HIIT Weeks 9-12
Do each exercise in the circuit for 40 seconds intensely and then slowly for 20 seconds.
Each individual exercise within the circuit should be done for 1 minute.

Follow the 1 minute **Warm Up** routine before commencing each HIIT session, never work out cold muscles.
This will start to get the blood pumping and can assist by loosening up your joints.
It will also help to reduce the risk of injury.

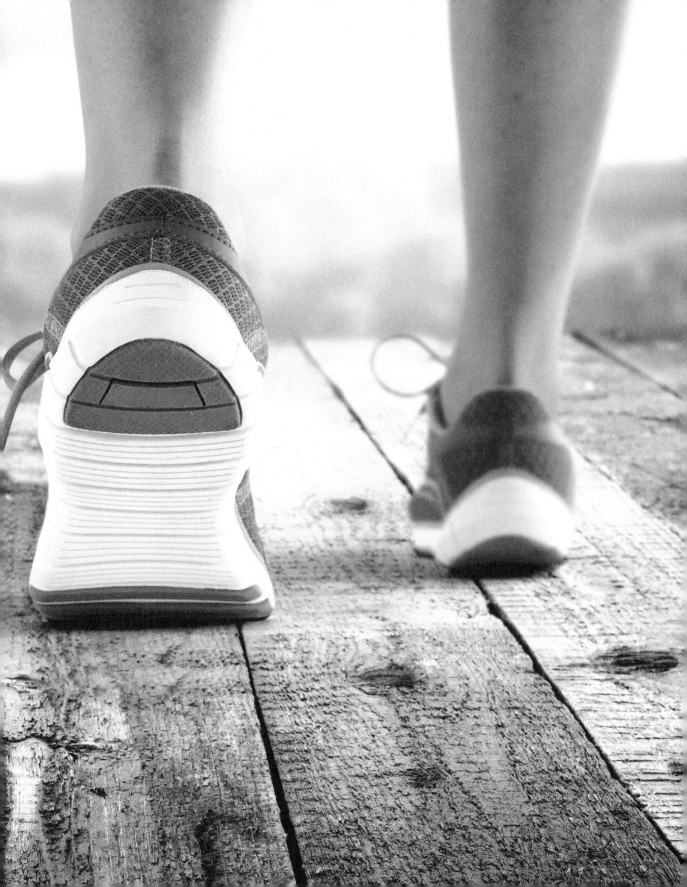

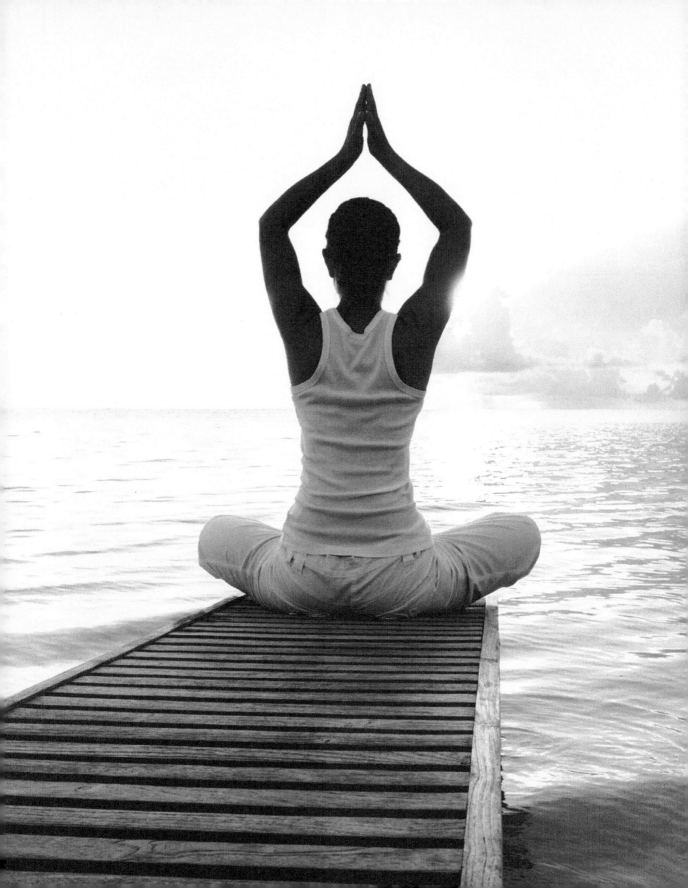

Included as well is a set of Yoga and Pilates type stretches designed to help you relax your muscles after the period of intense exercise. Always take at least 5 minutes or so after your HIIT session to perform these stretches - they will help to improve your flexibility and help to prevent soreness the next day.

To have an effective and successful exercise regime it is important to mix things up to add variety to your routine.
Other activities will accelerate your results, such as playing a ball sport, swimming, cycling or skiing.

Another great idea is to use technology. One of the best examples of this is Vibration training. It consists of either a disc or a plate which produces a pivoting or oscillating motion much like that of a see-saw or trampoline.
Exercising on a moving platform like this helps to work not only your core muscles but also your supporting stabilising muscles giving you a fuller body workout. This is called accelerated exercise and all you need to do is stand, sit or lean on the machine to get great results.

Incidental exercise can really assist with weight management and fitness goals. Try to walk more and to get the best results you can employ the principles of HIIT here as well - walk quickly for a minute then slower for 30 seconds and repeat.
It may also be a good idea to get a pedometer to count the number of steps that you are taking every day.

Poor dietary choices and little or no exercise is linked to weight gain and to many of the co-morbidities of obesity.

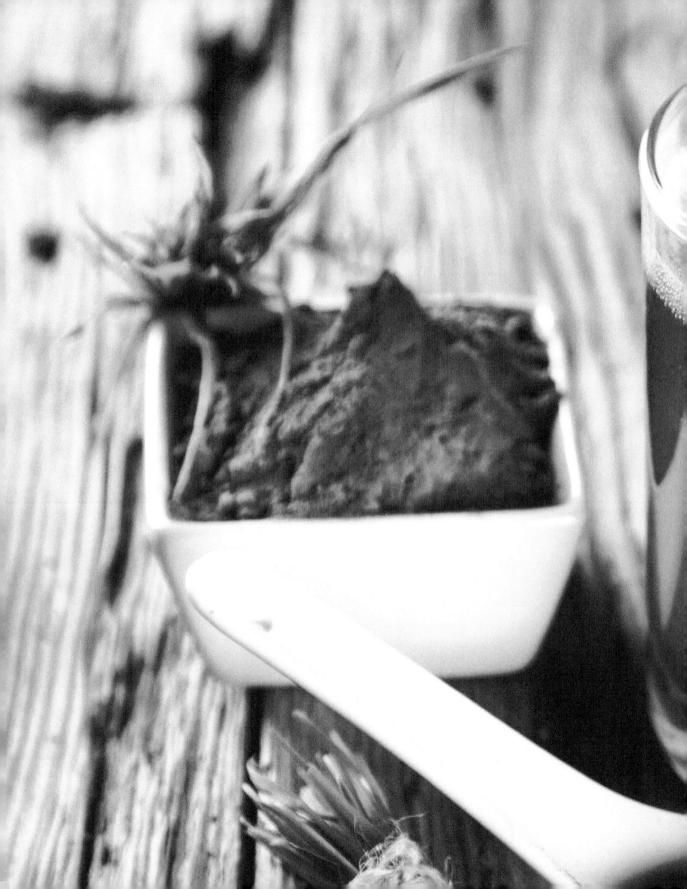

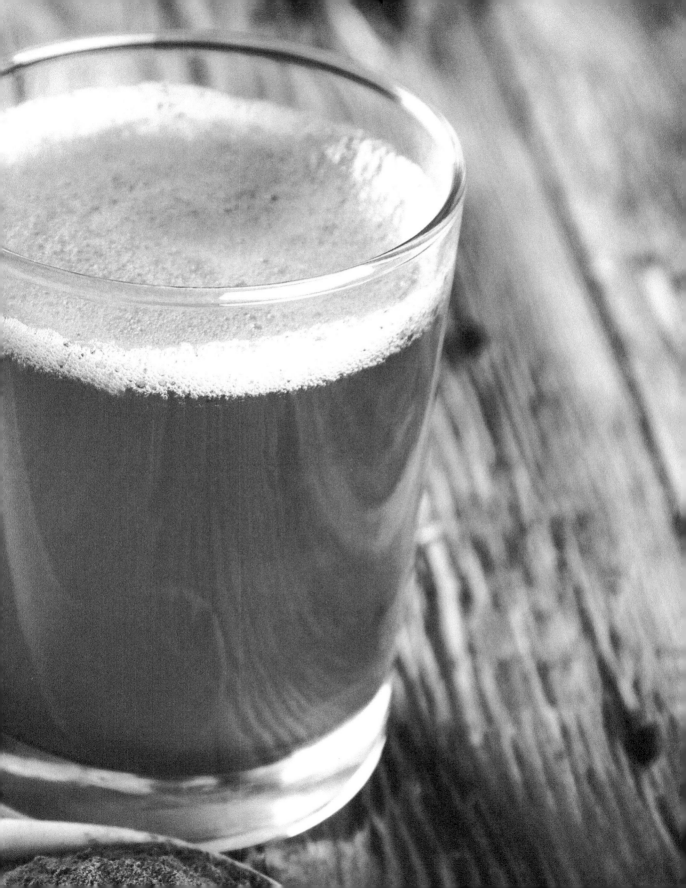

Intro Weeks 1 to 4

The first four weeks of the plan involve the consumption of predominately healthy plant based protein.
There are three main nutrient dense, low glycaemic meal choices together with vitamin rich snack options and healthy, delicious desserts.

There is also the option to replace certain meals or snacks with Sunwarrior Plant Based Protein shakes.
These are recommended to help kick start your metabolism and to help reduce cravings and unhealthy snacking. The plan includes healthy carbs to help with both cognition and energy levels.
Unlike many fad diets no one food group is excluded.

Wholefood supplements such as Go Figa, Go Green, Go Boost and Synergy Natural Organic Green Superfoods are recommended to help with alkalisation, digestion, satiety and cellular health.

Multi coloured fruits and vegatables are emphasised throughout in order to help keep antioxidant intake up and to assist weight loss results whilst helping to improve mood.

This section of the plan is designed to be immune boosting and to be protective at a cellular level whilst keeping energy levels up.
The emphasis is on improving digestive function in order to optimise nutritional outcomes.

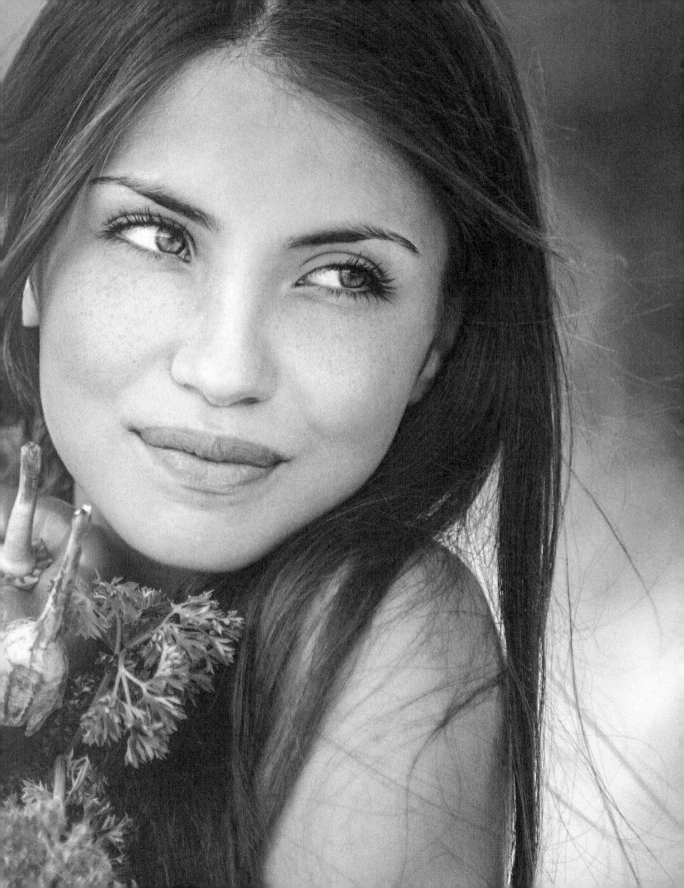

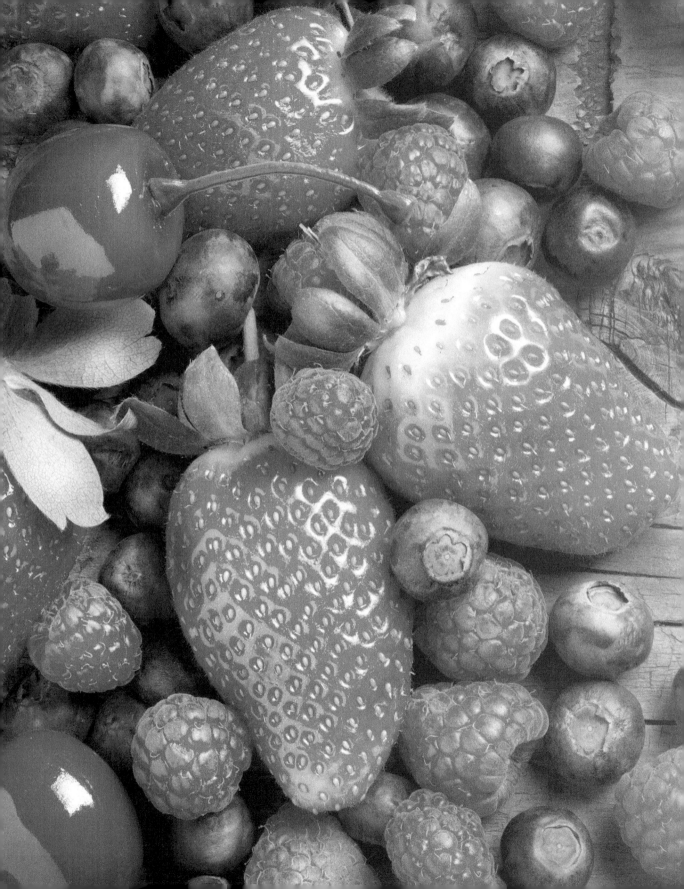

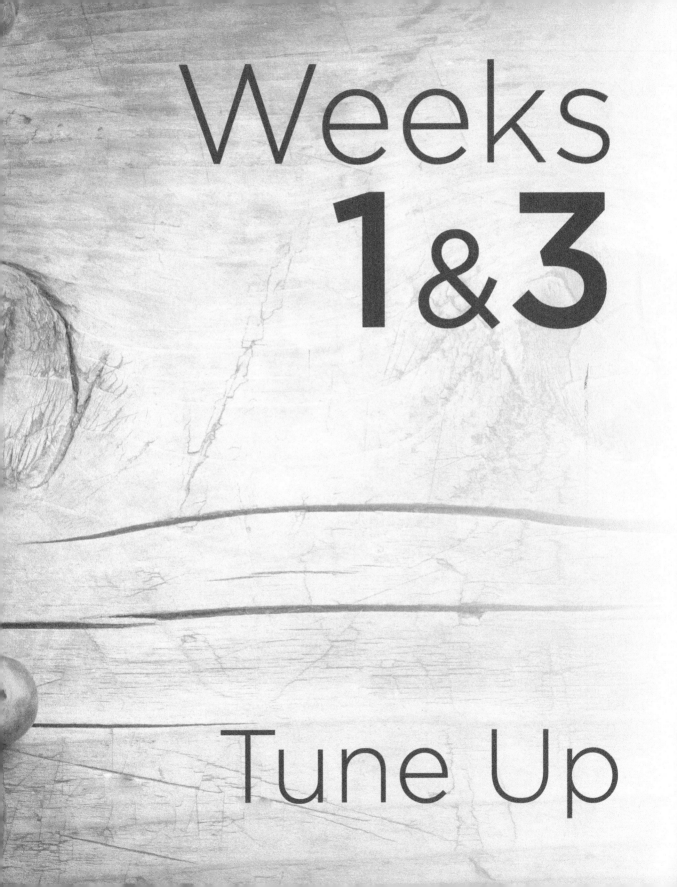

Weeks
1&3
Tune Up

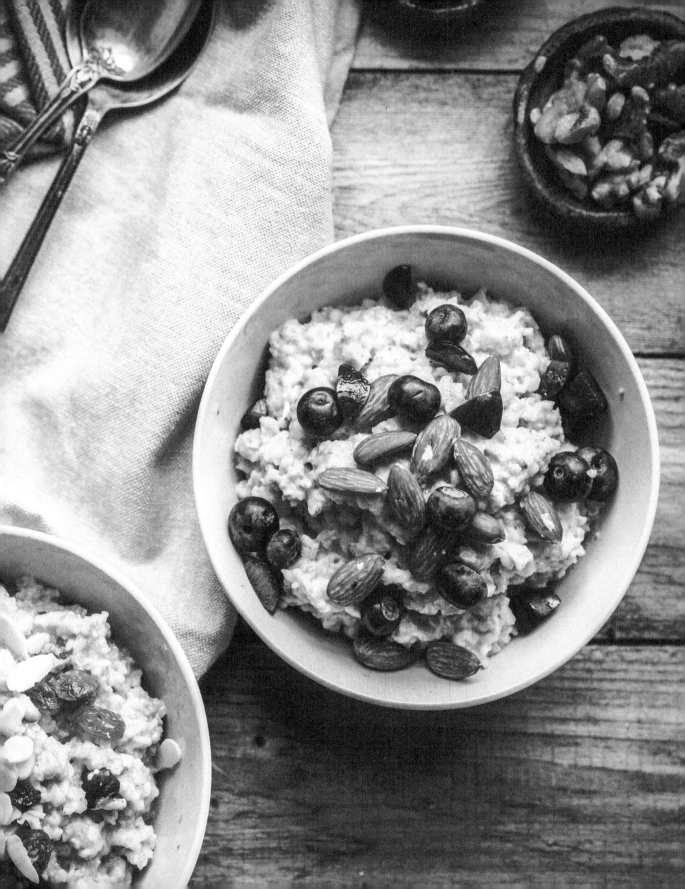

Before Breakfast

Lemon Blast

Half a glass of warm filtered water with the juice of half a lemon: to kick start the liver and gallbladder and digestive function. This is alkalising and helps with fat metabolism also.

Breakfast

Protein based to help with weight management; some carbs to provide energy to help with cognitive function:

Porridge with Berries

Add a few teaspoons of fresh or frozen berries to a small bowl of porridge with a dollop of unsweetened organic yogurt.

Berries are catabolic and help with fat burning and oats help to keep blood sugar levels stable which assist weight loss and mood.

OR

2 Organic or Free Range Eggs

Scrambled, Poached or Boiled and 1 piece of Rye or Wholegrain with Organic Butter or Olive oil Margarine.

OR

Banana Berry Smoothie

Blend 250 mls of rice or almond milk with 1 banana, or with a cup of berries, and a few almonds.

You can turbo charge your shake by adding 1 scoop of Plant Based Protein such as Sunwarrior - Natural, Vanilla or Chocolate.

These shakes can be used as a meal replacement as they are high in protein and amino acids that help to keep you feeling fuller for longer.

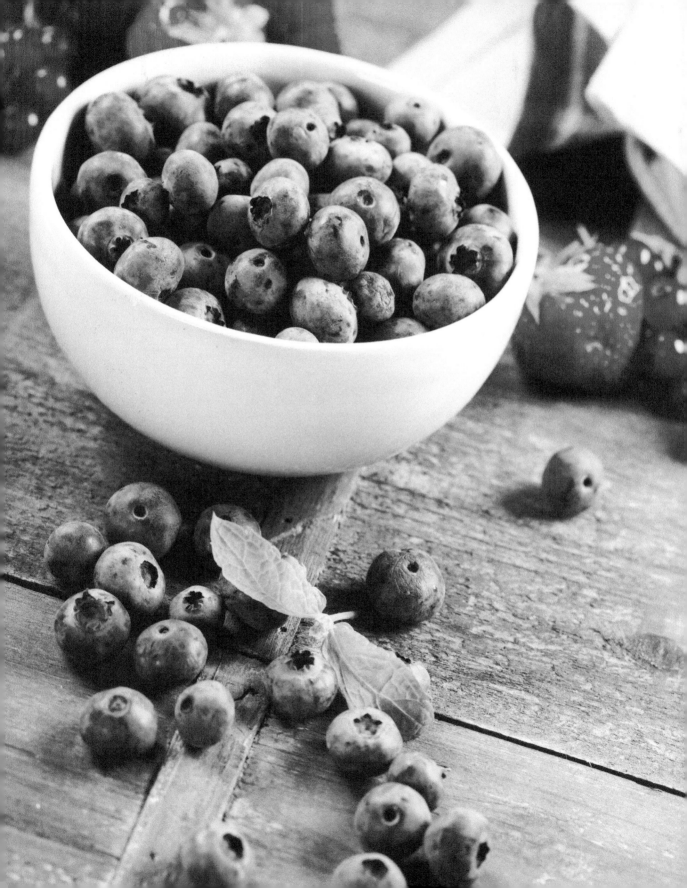

Mid Morning

Berry Bowl

To a small bowl of berries add a few almonds and organic unsweetened yogurt if desired.

Eating every few hours helps to control portion size and helps to regulate blood sugar levels helping to eliminate cravings.

OR

Apple with Almonds

1 Apple or other piece of fruit, as desired, with a few almonds.

OR

Yogurt

1 Small yogurt - choose unsweetened varieties like Natural or Greek Style with Honey.

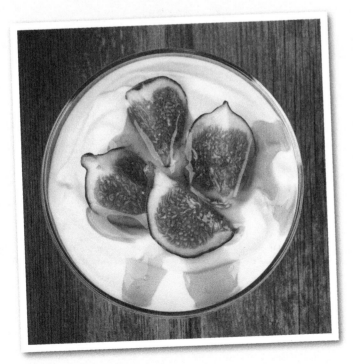

Before Lunch & Dinner
Spirulina Super Green Boost
6 Spirulina or Super Green tablets can be taken as they help with feelings of fullness and with controlling portion size.
They also help to alkalise the system.

Lunch

Broccoli, Cauliflower and Green Bean Soup

To 300 mls of water add a cupful of broccoli and of cauliflower and half a cup of green beans.

Simmer and season with fat burning thermogenic spices such as black pepper, cayenne, garlic or chilli.

OR

Grilled Salmon / Tofu or Tempeh

Grill 150g or less and serve with a cup of leafy greens.
Add an olive oil and balsamic vinegar dressing.

This is a protein based meal that is high in antioxidants and healthy omegas to help with mood and skin.

OR

Banana Berry Smoothie

Blend 250 mls of rice or almond milk with 1 banana or a cup of berries, and a few almonds.

You can turbo charge your shake by adding 1 scoop of Plant Based Protein such as Sunwarrior - Natural, Vanilla or Chocolate.

These shakes can be used as a meal replacement but only for one or two of the meals, not all three.

A half serve of the shake can be used as mid morning or mid afternoon snack - not if it is being used as a meal replacement though.

Mid Afternoon

Nut Butter Crispbread

Spread almond or cashew butter onto 1 or 2 crispbreads.

OR

Carrot and Celery Sticks

Serve with 50g of hummus.

OR

Avocado or Ricotta Crispbread

Add avocado or a thin spread of ricotta cheese to 1 or 2 crispbread slices.

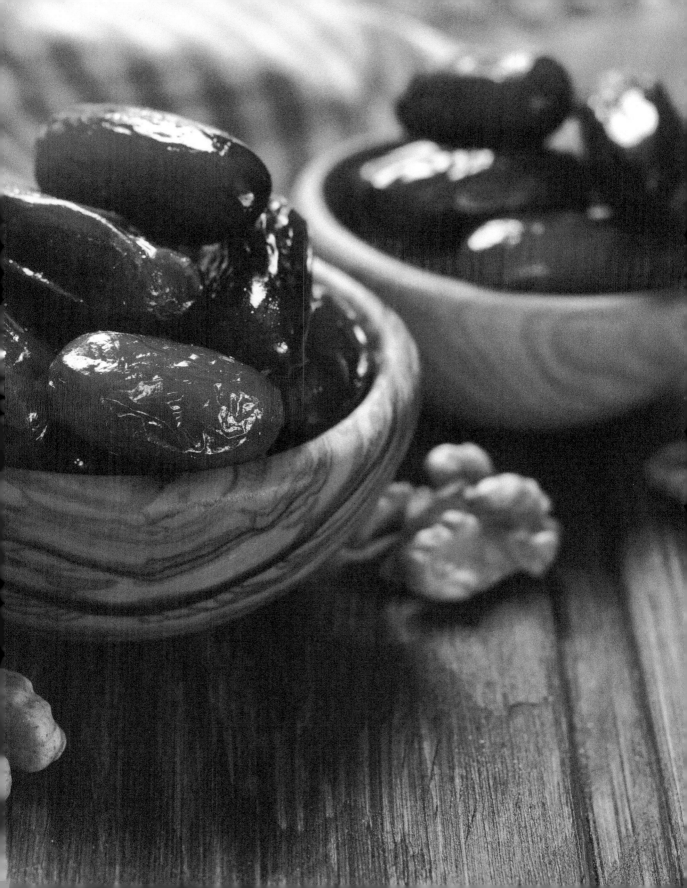

Dinner

Grilled Tuna / Tofu / Tempeh or Quorn

Grill a small piece, 150g or less, together with one to two cups of steamed green vegetables of choice.

The vegetables can be dressed with a little olive oil and garlic, sea salt or black pepper.

OR

2 to 3 Organic or Free Range Egg Omelette

Season with chilli or cayenne for thermogenic fat burning properties and serve with a cup of leafy greens.

OR

Green Vegetable and Cauliflower Stir Fry

Stir fry a cupful of green vegetables and cauliflower with a 100-150g protein option from dinner option 1.

Season with spices of choice.

Half a cup of brown rice can be added if desired.

After Dinner
Dates or Prunes with Rice or Almond Milk

2 or 3 Dates or prunes; served warm with a splash of unsweetened rice or almond milk.

Before Bed
Herbal Tea

1 Cup of herbal tea; choose calming varieties like chamomile, lemon balm or valerian.

Exercises for
Weeks 1&3

Warm Up
1 Minute Cardio - Jog

Start by 'walking on the spot' then take it into a jog.

After 30 seconds start to increase intensity and go as fast as you can, only taking your feet off the floor a couple of cms (or inches) and moving your arms fast as well until you hit the minute mark.

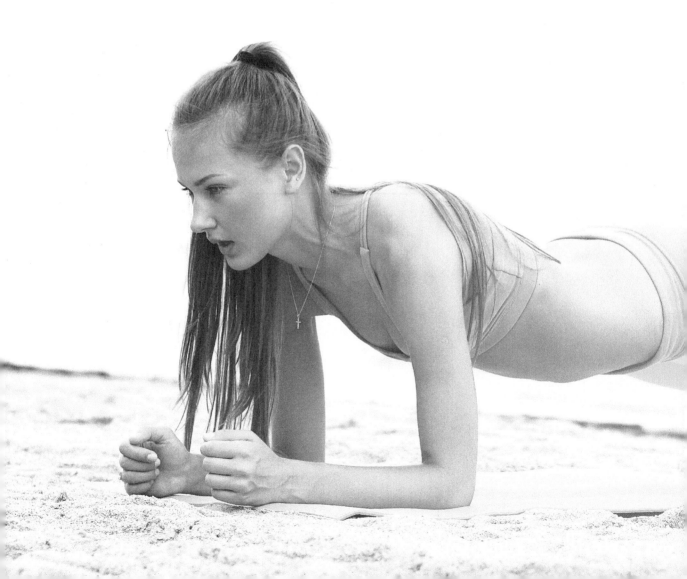

HIIT Circuit Weeks 1&3

Do each exercise in the circuit for 20 seconds intensely and then slowly for 40 seconds except for the Plank - this should be held for 20 seconds and then relaxed for 40 seconds at the beginner level.

Each individual exercise within the circuit should be done for 1 minute.

Beginner - complete once or twice
Intermediate - complete two or three times
Advanced - complete three or four times

Speed Squats

Stand with feet hip width apart and lower the hips down in a squat as if you're sitting on a low chair, sticking out your butt behind you.
Move quickly back to a standing position and repeat.

As you squat down keep arms straight but raise them to parallel with the floor as you squat down.

Keep the timing steady.

Plank

Start by getting into a push up position.

Beginners - on knees / elbows
Intermediate - on toes / hands
Advanced - move from elbows to hands and alternate from one to the other keeping the core activated at all times.

Bend your elbows and rest your weight onto your forearms or hands.

Engage your core by pulling your belly button in towards your spine.

To increase the intensity of the intermediate move, lift 1 leg by 5cms from the floor and then lower and change.
Alternate legs every 5 seconds.

Static Running

Assume 'Running Position', with one leg forward, one back - as if about to start a race.

Bend your arms and move them back and forth quickly as if you are running very fast.

Increase the speed of the movement to increase the intensity and to raise the heart rate.

Abs - Leg Raise & Touch Toes

Lie on your back with your shoulders on the floor and your legs straight up in the air.

Breathe in.

As you exhale reach your hands towards toes, lifting shoulders away from the ground.

Touch your toes if possible and pulse.

Stretch & Relax

Seated forward bend. (Yoga - 'Paschimottanasana').

Sit down with your legs flat and straight out in front of you.

Breathe in, raise hands to the ceiling and slowly lean forward keeping your back straight initially.

Hold this position reaching as far towards your toes as you can.

Either hold hands around your feet, or use a small towel around your feet to draw yourself further into the stretch.

Aim to hold this position for 1 minute, or longer.

Instructional videos available at **www.superfoodist.com**

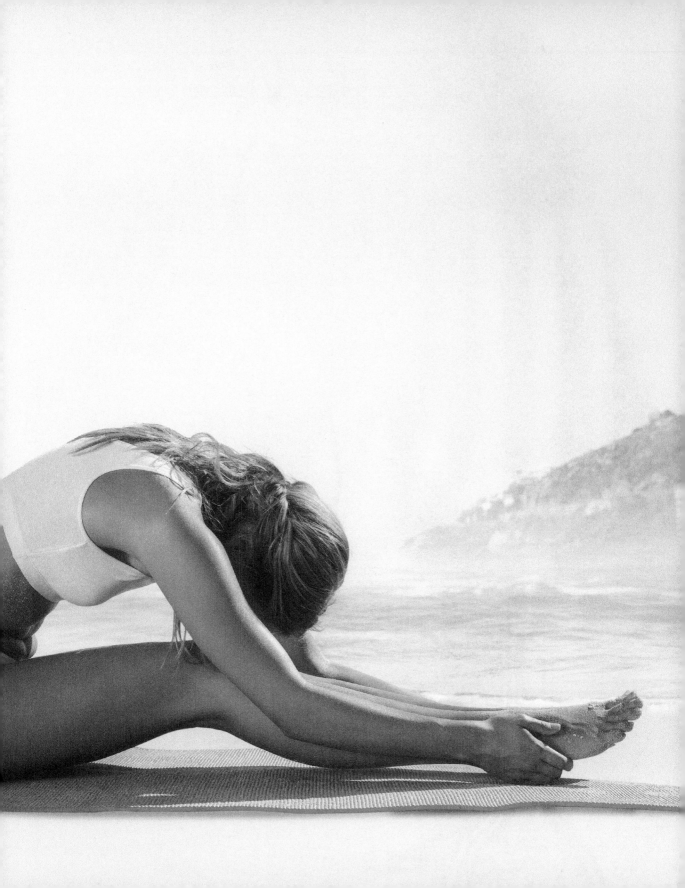

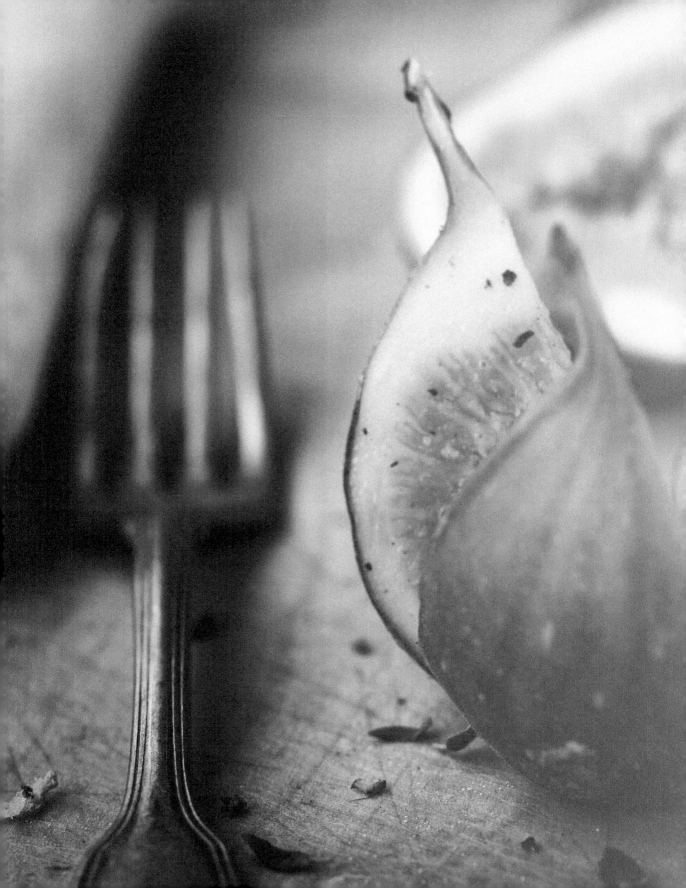

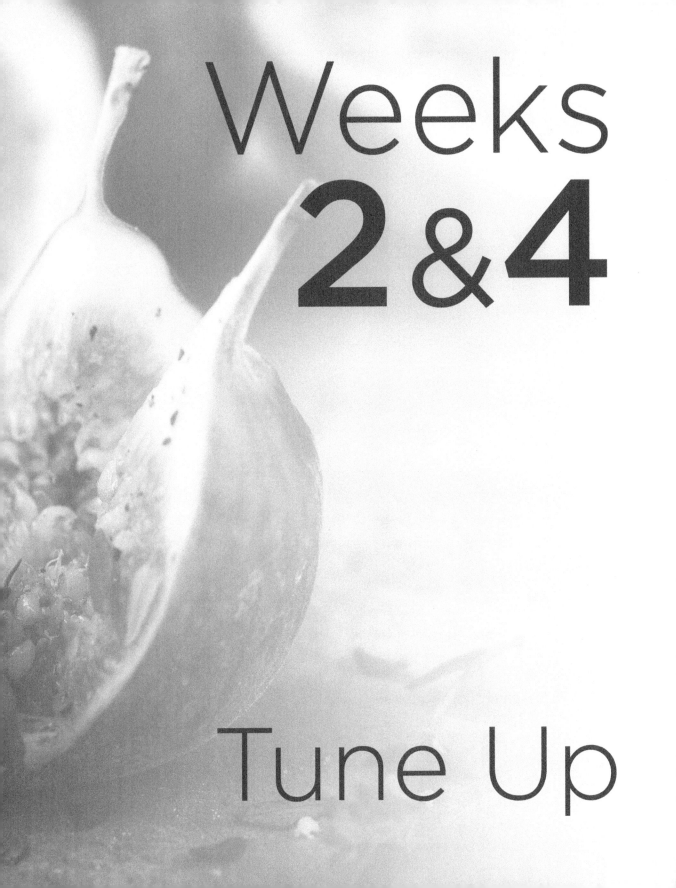

Weeks
2&4

Tune Up

Before Breakfast
Grapefruit Blast

Half a glass of warm filtered water with the juice of half a grapefruit to kick start the liver and gallbladder and digestive function.

This early morning combination helps with fat metabolism also.

Breakfast

Poached Organic or Free Range Eggs with Smoked Tofu or Salmon

2 Poached or scrambled eggs; with a palm sized piece of grilled smoked salmon or tofu.

OR

Carrot, Apple and Ginger Juice

250 mls of store bought cold pressed juice.

This fruit and vegetable mix is high in phytonutrients and enzymes for anti ageing cellular health.

Ginger is a circulatory, digestive and immune system tonic.

Have with a handful of pumpkin seeds, almonds, cashews or walnuts to boost protein and vitamin content.

The seeds and nuts also assist with satiety and will help to reduce cravings throughout the day.

OR

Banana and Berry Smoothie

Blend or blast 250 mls of unsweetened rice or almond milk with 1 banana, or with a cup of berries, and a few almonds.

You can boost your shake by adding 1 scoop of Plant Based Protein such as Sunwarrior - Natural, Vanilla or Chocolate.

These shakes can be used as a meal replacement as they are high in protein and amino acids that help to keep you feeling fuller for longer whilst providing energy.

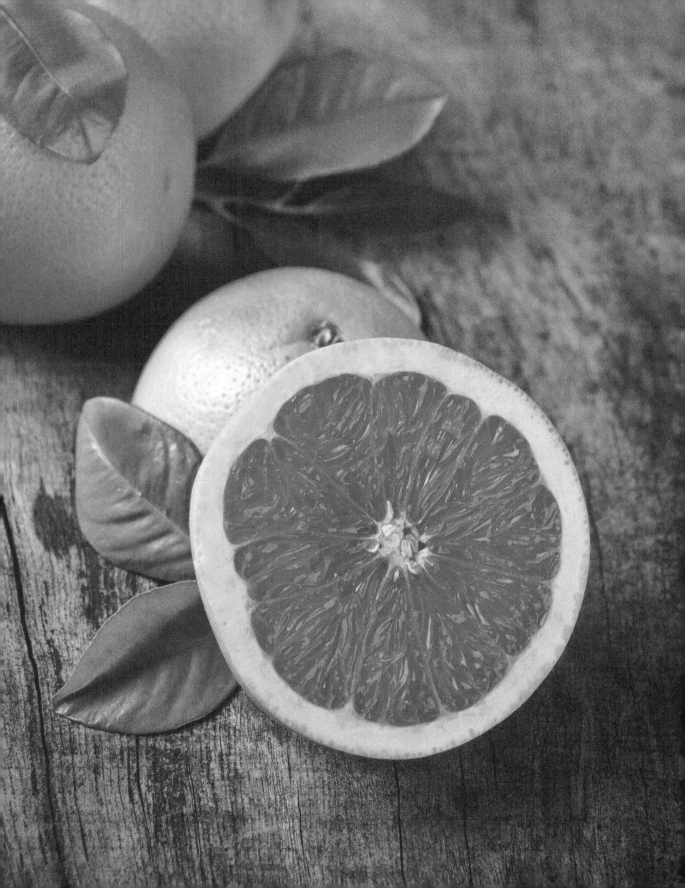

Mid Morning

Fruit and Nuts Yogurt Treat

1 Banana or apple; with a few almonds and a few teaspoons of yogurt if desired.

Eating every few hours helps to control portion size and helps to regulate blood sugar levels thereby reducing cravings and helping with mood and cognitive performance.

OR

Cashew Nut Fruit Bowl

1 Small bowl portion of fruit salad; with a few cashew nuts. Berries, apples, pears and melons are recommended.

OR

Brown Rice Cakes

2 Rice cakes with avocado or nut butter - almond or cashew preferably.
This snack is rich in antioxidants and healthy omegas.

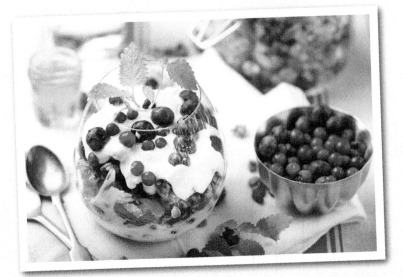

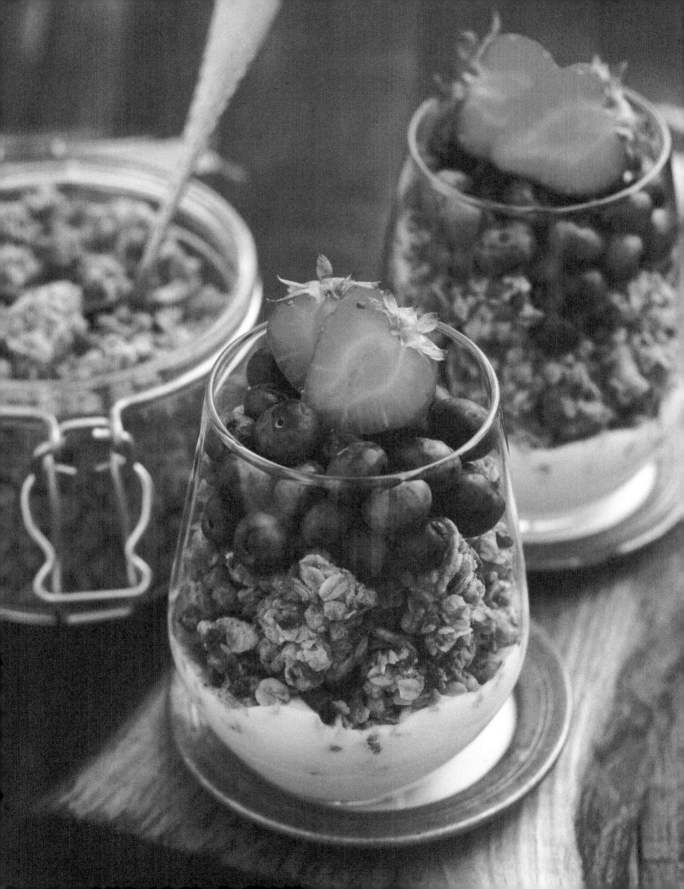

Before Lunch & Dinner

Spirulina Super Green Boost

6 Spirulina or Super Green tablets can be taken as they help with feelings of fullness and with controlling portion size.

They also help to alkalise and detox the system.

Lunch

Grilled Tofu / Quorn / Salmon / Tuna / Tempeh

Grill 150g or less of one of the above protein choices.

Serve with a cup of chilli chick peas and mixed beans - add a teaspoon of olive oil, balsamic vinegar and a little chilli or cayenne to the chick peas.

This protein based meal is high in antioxidants to boost immunity and is rich in healthy omegas to help with mood, cognition and skin conditions.

OR

Banana & Berry Smoothie

Smoothie as per breakfast.

These smoothies can be used as a meal replacement but only for one or two of the meals, not for all three.

A half serve size can be used as mid morning or mid afternoon snack but not if it is being used as a meal replacement though.

OR

Spinach, Bean and Lentil Soup

Add 4 tablespoons in total of mixed beans and lentils and two generous handfuls of spinach to 300 mls of water, and bring slowly to the boil.

Season with thermogenic spices such as black pepper, garlic, cayenne, garlic or chilli.

A high protein lunch option that will assist with regularity.

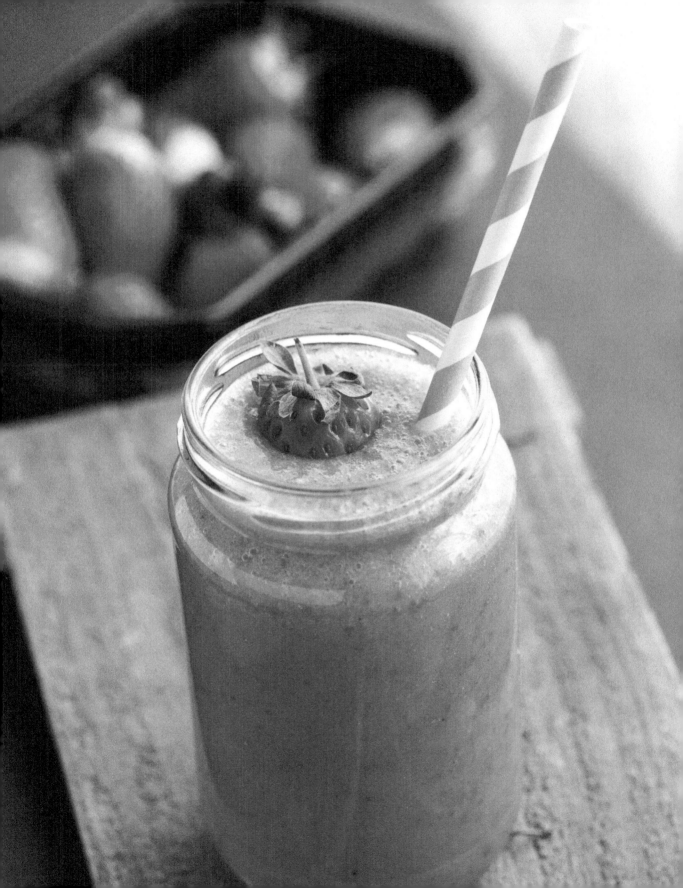

Mid Afternoon

Date or Prune Nut Mix

4 or 5 Dried dates or prunes; with 2 or 3 teaspoons of mixed nuts or seeds.

OR

Seeds, Nuts and Apple

2 or 3 Teaspoons of mixed nuts and seeds with half an apple.

OR

Yogurt

1 Small unsweetened Natural or Greek Style yogurt.

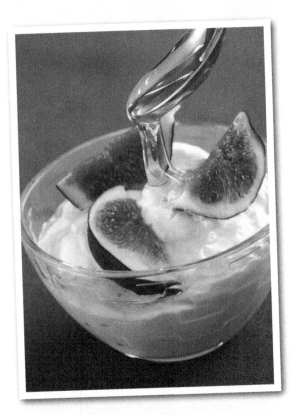

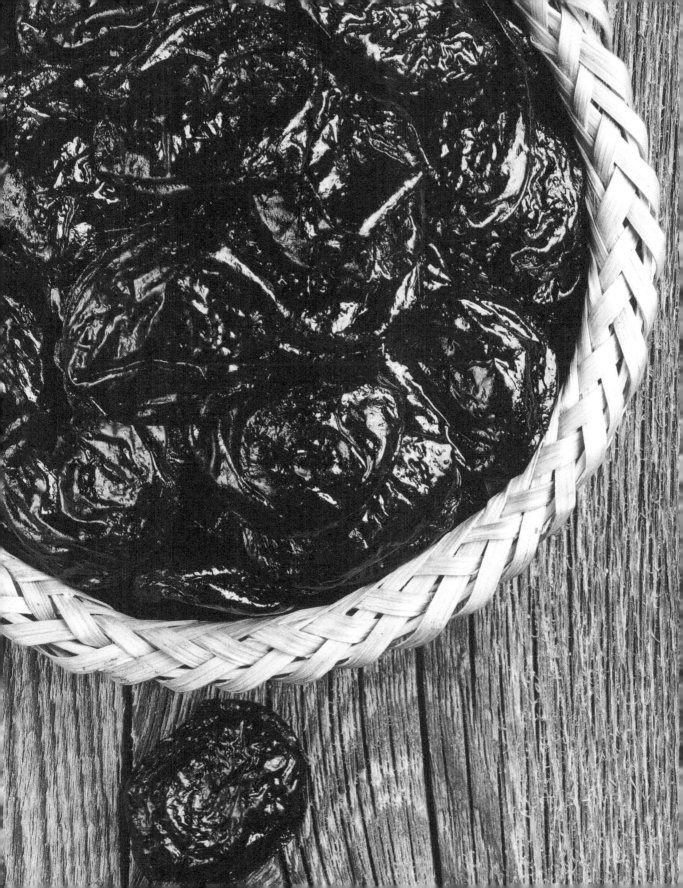

Dinner

Lightly Fried Tofu / Quorn / Tempeh with Steamed Greens

Lightly fry 150g or less of one of these protein options.

Serve together with a cup or two of green steamed vegetables.

Season with thermogenic spices such as cayenne, chilli, garlic or black pepper.

Fry on a low heat using a little cold pressed olive oil.

OR

Chilli Omelette with Salad or Green Beans

2 to 3 Organic or free range eggs seasoned with chilli or cayenne for their thermogenic properties.

Serve with a small cup of salad greens or steamed green beans.

OR

Broccoli, Green Beans and Spinach Stir Fry

Together with the protein choice from dinner option 1 stir fry a cupful of broccoli and one of green beans in olive oil.

Season with spices of choice and serve with half a cup of brown rice.

After Dinner

Cacao / Cocoa Milk

Warm a cup of unsweetened rice or almond milk slowly.

Add a teaspoon of 100% raw cacao or cocoa and a hint of chilli powder to help burn fat if desired.

Before Bed

Herbal Tea

1 Cup of herbal tea; choose calming varieties like chamomile, lemon balm or valerian to hydrate and soothe.

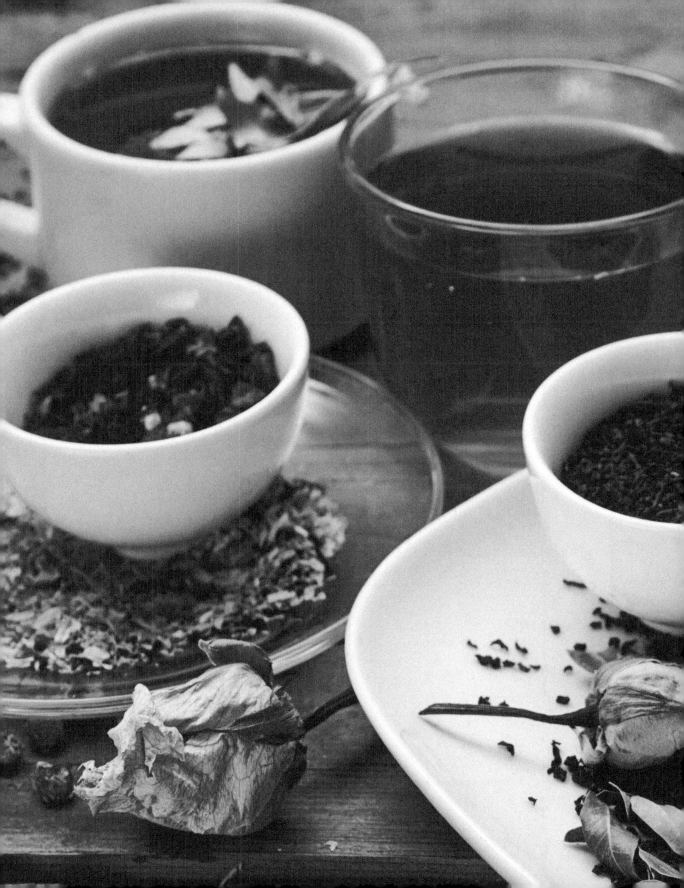

Exercises for
Weeks 2 & 4

Warm Up
1 Minute Cardio - Knee Raise

Hold your hands out in front of you and lift your knees toward your hands one at a time, then take it into a jog and raise the hands until they are parallel to the floor, touching your knees to your hands if possible.

To increase intensity increase the speed and the height of the knees.

To engage the oblique muscles (side core) more go back to a walking speed.

Take your knee toward the opposite elbow with your hands placed behind your head and alternate.

HIIT Circuit Weeks 2&4

Do each exercise in the circuit for 20 seconds intensely and then slowly for 40 seconds.
Each individual exercise within the circuit should be done for 1 minute.

Beginner - complete once or twice
Intermediate - complete two or three times
Advanced - complete three or four times

Superman

Come down onto all fours.

Activate core by drawing in the belly button towards the spine.

Stretch forward your right arm, and outstretch your left leg, keeping them parallel to the floor, hold for 5 seconds then repeat with your opposite arm and leg till you reach your chosen time level.

Mountain Climbers

Assume a high Plank position (on hands and toes)

Make sure the shoulders are positioned over the wrists.

From here draw one knee at a time towards the nose and return to the start position.

Perform this movement quickly as if you were 'running'.
Keep the hips low.

To activate the oblique muscles (side core) take the knee toward the opposite elbow as you move it forward.

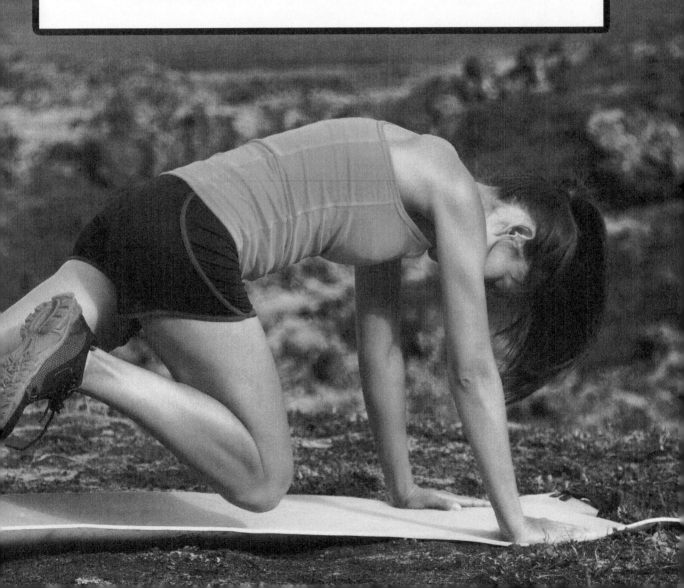

Squat with Shoulder Press

Just hands only or light weights.

Start in a standing position and go down to a low squat with your hands at shoulder level and with your arms outstretched to the side keeping your elbows bent.

As you stand, move the hands (with weights) straight up overhead.

Squat and repeat.

Abs - Elbow to Knee (Obliques)

Slow motion.

Lying down, raise your lower legs to a tabletop position (lower legs parallel to floor), with your hands held behind supporting your head.

Rotate your elbow to the opposite knee as you stretch out the other leg and Repeat.

Keep your shoulders off the floor at all times to engage the abdominals.

Stretch & Relax

Child's Pose' (Yoga - 'Balasana').

Sit on your heels and place your knees either together or apart (i.e. towards the edge of your yoga mat).

Sitting back onto your heels walk your hands forwards.

Keep your bottom on your heels and stretch out placing the forearms on the mat ahead of you.

Lower your head to the mat.

This primarily stretches your lower back, hips and knees.

Hold for at least 1 minute.

Instructional videos available at **www.superfoodist.com**

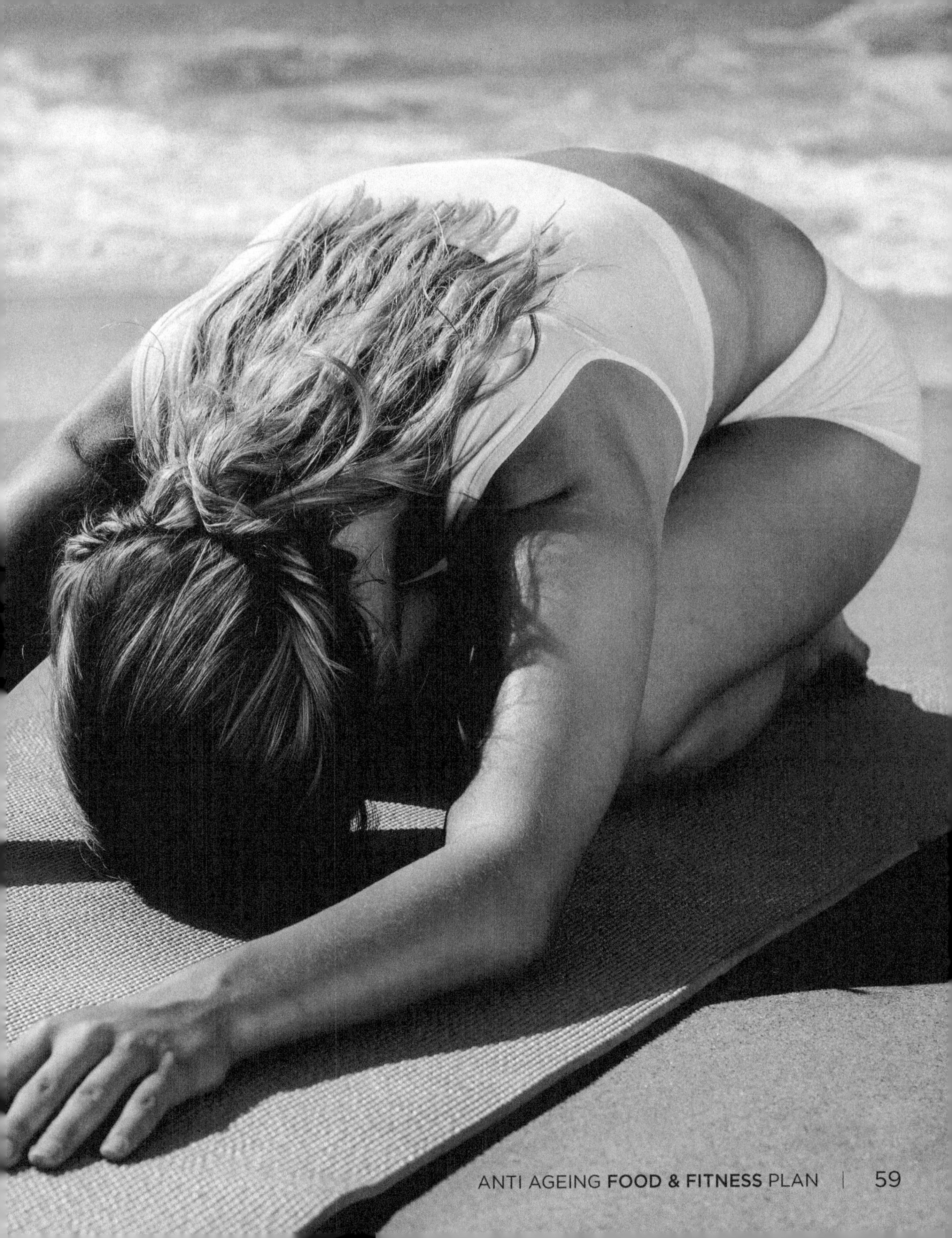

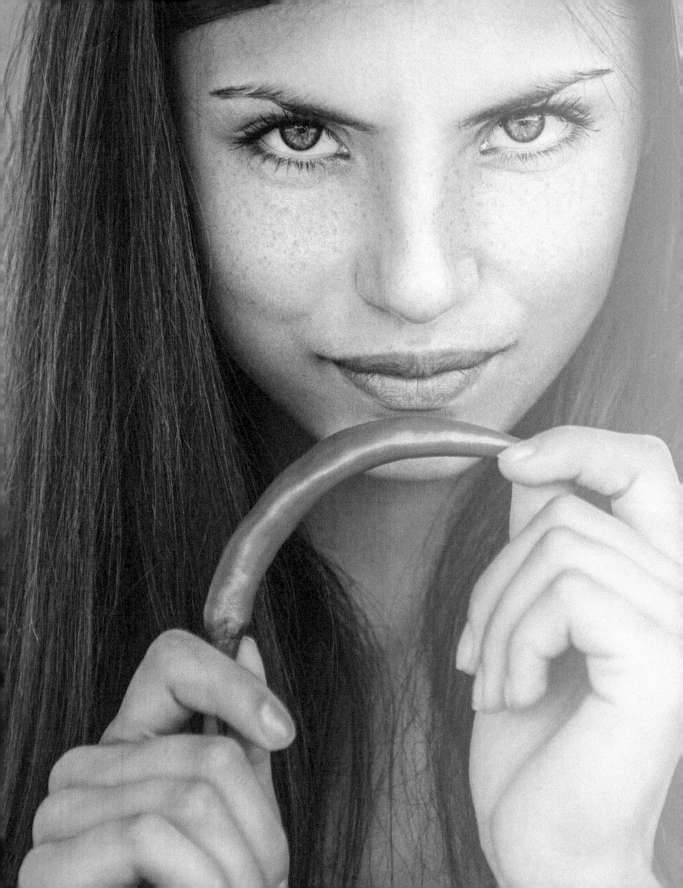

intro Weeks 5 to 8

During weeks 5 to 8 the plan alters slightly to include more thermogenic spices such as cayenne, chilli, pepper and turmeric in order to more effectively assist with the metabolism of fat from the body.

Blood sugar regulating super spice, cinnamon, is also recommended throughout this four week period to help reduce cravings and to assist with weight management.

Weeks 5 to 8 of the plan are not all that different from the initial four weeks however, one thing that you will note is that breakfast is now recommended to be solely a protein shake or smoothie.
This will really get your metabolism going for the day and help with weight management.

Do not skip breakfast as this will lead to a slow down in your metabolic rate and make it harder for you to lose weight. Skipping breakfast also puts more pressure on the nervous system and will result in your body producing more adrenaline and cortisol - high levels of these two hormones make it harder biochemically for your body to metabolise fat and can lead to increased weight around the tummy area.
This visceral fat accumulation is also an increased cardiovascular risk.

When a juice is recommended, if you do not have a juicer, make sure that any juice that is store bought is cold pressed.
Always have a vegetable and fruit juice combination as this lowers the glycaemic load - a lower GL regulates blood sugar better.
Straight fruit juice can be too high in natural sugars and can cause unwanted blood sugar spikes.

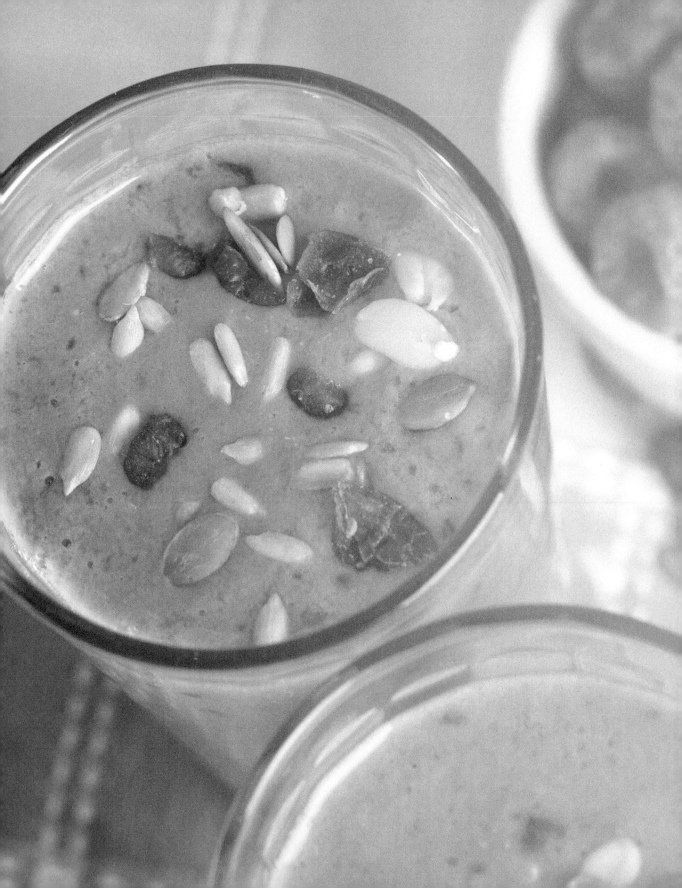

Weeks
5&7

Rev Up

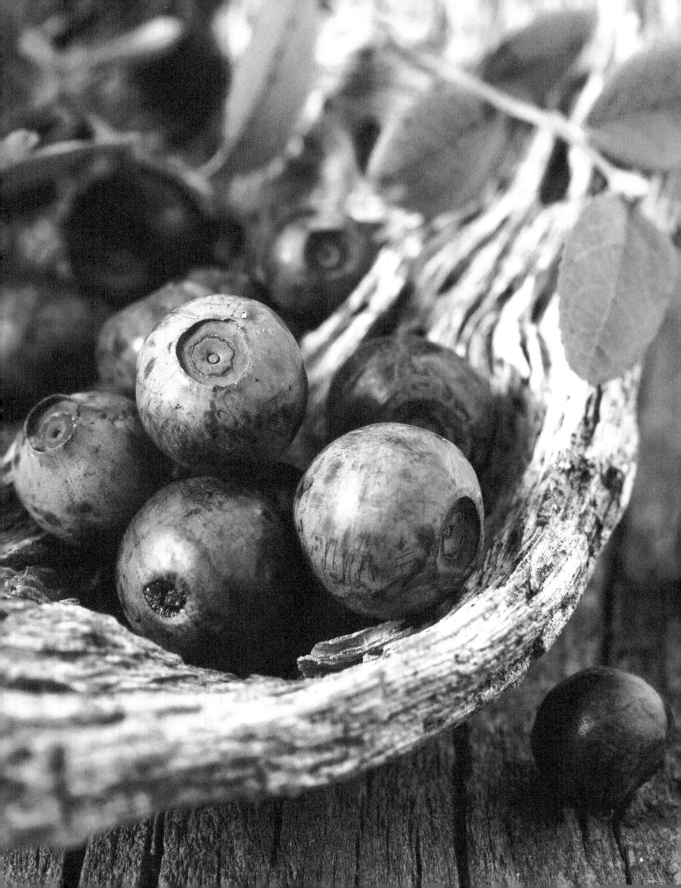

Before Breakfast
Lemon Blast

Half a glass of warm filtered water with the juice of half a lemon.
This will kickstart the liver and gallbladder and assist with digestive function.

Add a teaspoon of cinnamon to help reduce cravings and steady mood.

Breakfast
Blueberry Protein Smoothie

Blend or blast 1 scoop of Plant Based Protein Powder like Sunwarrior Vanilla with 250mls of unsweetened rice or almond milk and a cup of blueberries.
Add 7 or 8 almonds to increase satiety if desired.

This nutritional blast is now used as a meal replacement.
It is high in protein and amino acids to help keep you fuller for longer and will assist in energy production.

A handful of spinach can also be used to increase magnesium levels.
One teaspoon of Go Figa - Superfood Fig powder can also be included to increase nutrient density and satiety.

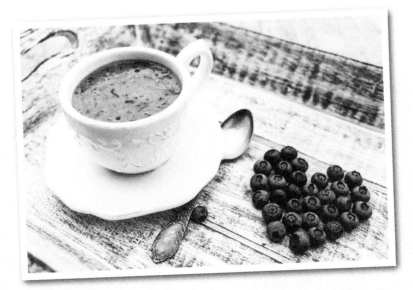

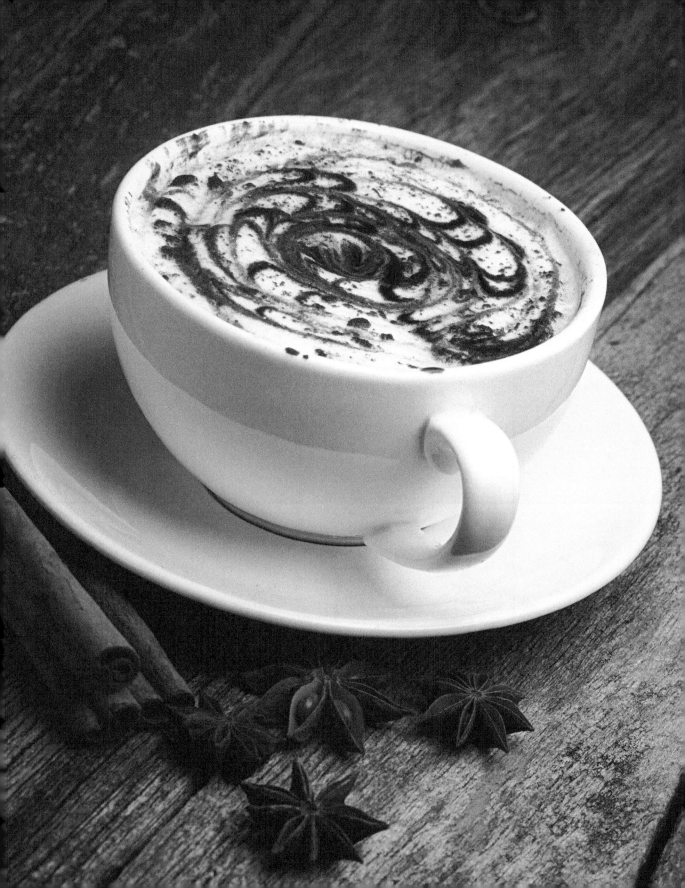

Mid Morning

Seasonal Small Nutty Fruit Bowl

Top a small bowl of seasonal fruit with 5 or 6 almonds or cashews.

Can be served with a dollop of unsweetened organic yogurt.

The fruit and nuts are nutrient dense and help with both cognitive and immune function - the nuts provide protein to help with fullness.

OR

Apple and Pecans

1 Apple with 6 to 8 pecans.

OR

Omega Density Juice

Blend or blast 7 cashews or almonds with 1 teaspoon of chia seeds, linseeds and sesame seeds.

Add 1 cup of leafy greens and half an avocado and half a banana.

Add a glass of water or coconut water.

This immune booster is high in phytonutrients and is packed full of enzymes for anti ageing cellular health.

The seeds are rich in healthy omegas to promote hair, skin and nail health.

These omegas also assist with cognitive function and weight management.

This option is particularly filling so you will need a smaller lunch portion.

OR

Coffee, Tea or Dandelion Tea

1 Cup of coffee or tea if desired.

This is a great time of day to maximise the fat burning qualities of caffeine.

Do not sweeten with sugar or artificial sweeteners - use half a teaspoon of honey or stevia if necessary.

The dandelion tea option is good to help reduce bloating and fluid retention.

It also stimulates liver function.

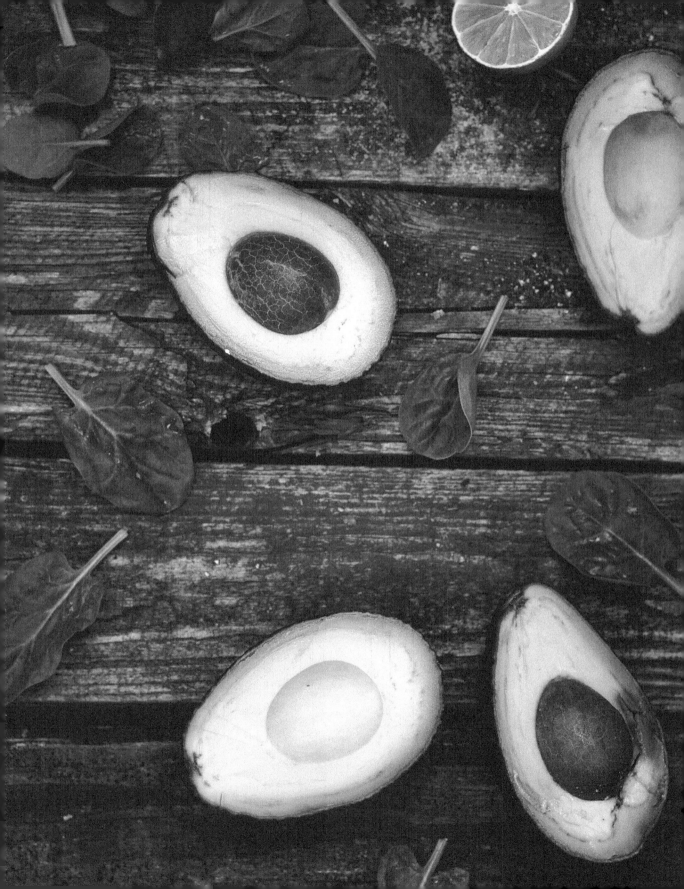

Before Lunch & Dinner

Spirulina Super Green Boost

6 Spirulina or Super Green tablets can be taken as they help with feelings of fullness and control portion size - they also help to alkalise the system.

Lunch

Avocado Scrambled Eggs

2 or 3 Organic or free range scrambled eggs with half an avocado. Season with chilli, cayenne or black pepper.

OR

Tofu with Salad Greens

A small bowl of lightly fried tofu - fry slowly using cold pressed olive oil.

Serve with a cup sized portion of asparagus, salad greens and broccoli together with 3 or 4 small tomatoes.

Add olive oil, balsamic vinegar and fresh cracked black pepper.

The salad is rich in enzymes with the vinegar and black pepper promotes fat burning - the olive oil provides a good source of healthy omegas.

OR

Avocado and Black Pepper Crispbread

Top 2 or 3 crispbreads with half an avocado and black pepper.

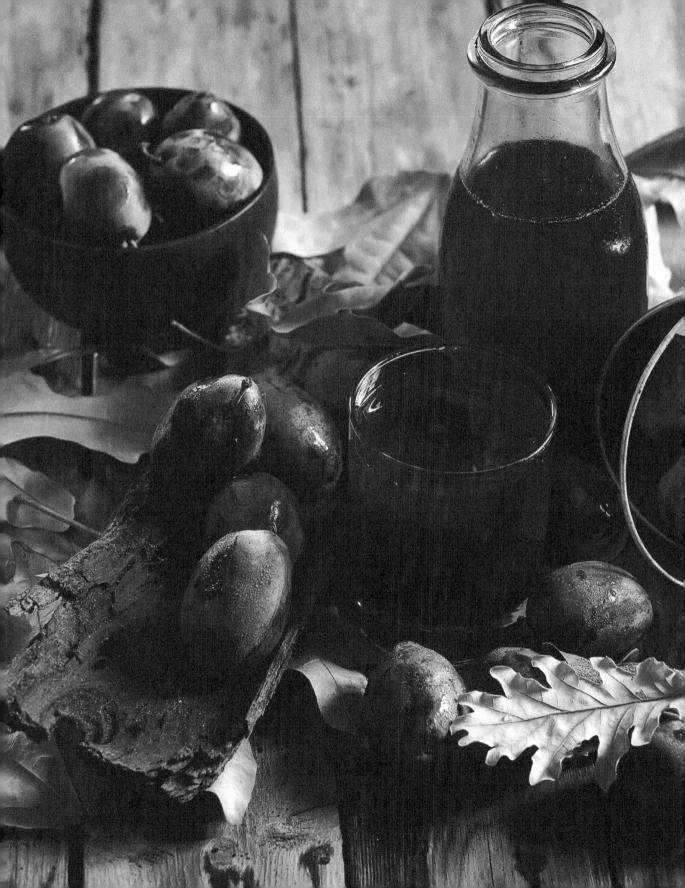

Mid Afternoon

Prune Snack with Nuts

3 or 4 Prunes or a glass of unsweetened organic prune juice with one banana.

If you're constipated it's harder to lose weight so regularity is important.

This snack is a great help with energy - both physical and mental. Have with 2 teaspoons of mixed nuts and seeds for protein to help keep you satisfied till dinner.

OR

Pecan / Walnut Fruit Bowl

Small mixed fruit bowl with 6 or 7 pecans or walnuts - any combination of fruits although berries are best.

OR

Peppermint or Spearmint Tea

One cup of peppermint or spearmint tea - to calm and stimulate digestion.

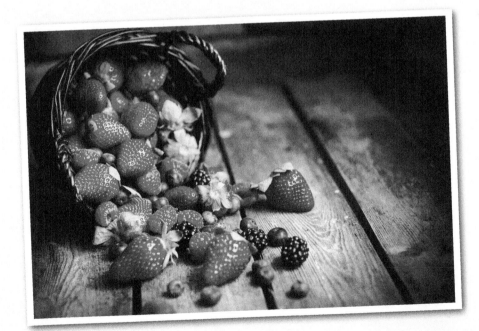

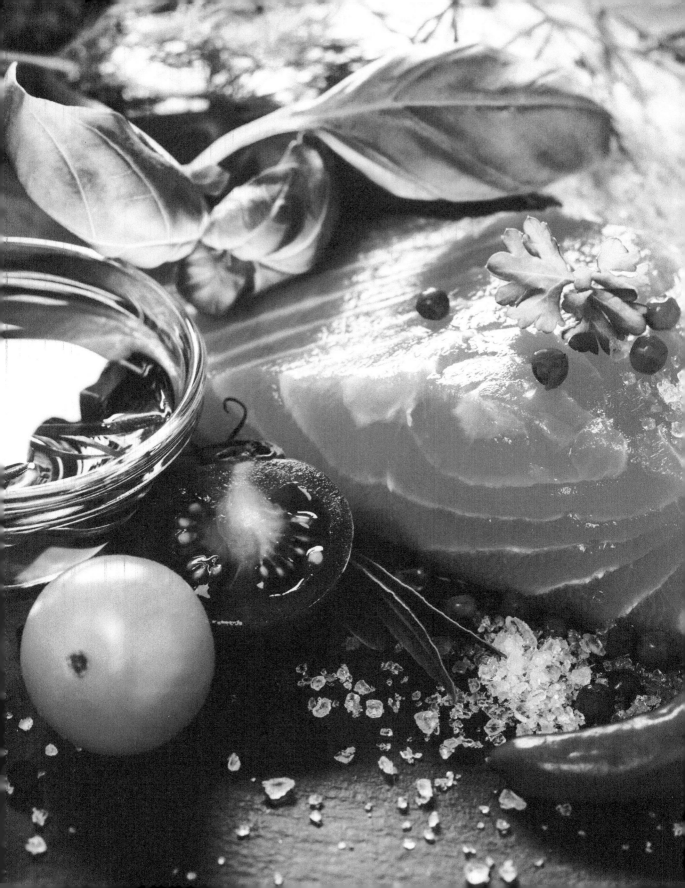

Dinner

Grilled Tofu or Salmon with Salad

Grill a small piece of tofu or salmon, 100 - 150g.

Serve with a bowl of salad green leaves dressed with olive oil, cracked black pepper and sea salt.

OR

Cashew and Pine Nut Vegetable Stir Fry

Stir fry 2 cups of a vegetable medley of your choice in cold pressed olive oil.

When ready add 5 or 6 cashews and a handful of pine nuts.

Make sure you add spices to taste as they stimulate the digestive process and speed up metabolism - use soy sauce, ginger, chilli and garlic.

Can be served with a small cup of brown rice.

OR

Grilled Kebabs

Thread small chunks of tuna, salmon or tofu and alternate with veggies such as broccoli, peppers and mushrooms onto a skewer and cook as preferred.

Serve on a bed of lettuce.

Season with spices of choice.

AND

Dandelion Tea / Coffee

1 Cup of herbal tea, such as unsweetened dandelion, fennel, fenugreek or liquorice.

Dandelion's bitter qualities aid liver function making it good for weight loss, fluid retention, bloating and skin conditions.

Fennel and fenugreek are both digestive tonics whilst liquorice is an adrenal tonic and energy booster.

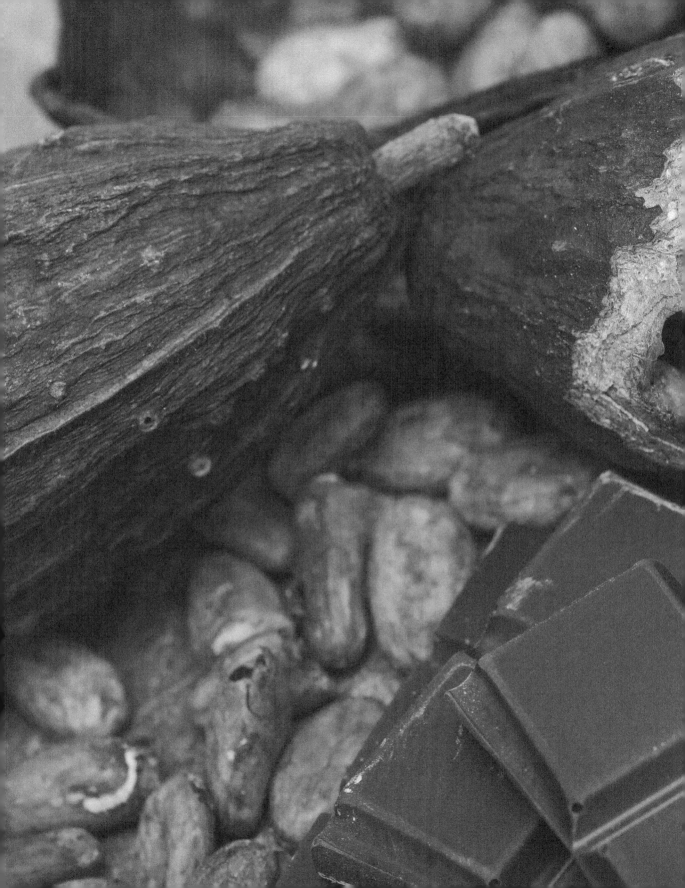

After Dinner

Cacao treat

1 Teaspoon of cacao with 250mls of unsweetened rice or almond milk.
This can be served hot or cold and sweetened with a little honey.
Have with a handful of nuts and dried fruits if desired as they will help to
stabilise mood and satisfy a sweet tooth.
Half a teaspoon of chilli powder can be added to help with lymphatic
function and fat burning.

OR

Dark Chocolate Squares and Almonds

2 Squares of 75% or greater dark chocolate and 5 or 6 almonds.

Before Bed

Calming Herbal Tea

1 Cup of herbal tea - choose a calming variety like chamomile,
lemon balm or valerian.
Sweet dreams!

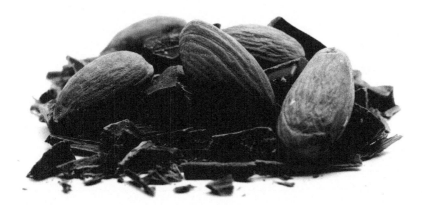

Exercises for
Weeks 5&7

Warm Up
1 Minute Cardio - Glute Reverse Kicks

Start in a jog, then place your hands behind your back at waist level, palms facing out and begin to kick your heels into your hands - for approx 30 seconds.

Change direction and place your arms out in front of you and start to kick your feet toward the opposite hand - again for 30 seconds and try to touch your toes.

HIIT Circuit Weeks 5&7

Do each exercise in the circuit for 30 seconds intensely and then slowly for 30 seconds except for the Side Plank - this should be held for 30 seconds and then relaxed for 30 seconds.
Each individual exercise within the circuit should be done for 1 minute.

Beginner - complete once or twice
Intermediate - complete two or three times
Advanced - complete three or four times

Lunge with Bicep Curl
Start standing straight.

Take one big step forward lowering your back knee to the ground taking your front knee over the ankle as you perform a bicep curl.

Push back to standing and alternate legs.

Don't take your knee past your ankle.

Side Plank

Lie on your side then place your hand on the floor, directly under your shoulder, and raise your body to a Plank (straight) position.

If you have issues with your wrists, this can be done on your elbow.

Hold this static pose for half of your allotted time frame, then turn and do the opposite side.

To increase the intensity do small pulsing movements raising the hips toward the ceiling - only by about 5 cms or 2 1/2 inches.

Burpee / Jump back then stand

Start in standing position.

Take your hands flat to the floor assuming a crouch position.

Jump the legs back to a high Plank pose then return to standing and repeat.

To increase intensity do an actual Burpee, where you jump in the air (rather then just going to a standing position) and add in a push up in place of one of the jump backs.

Abs - Heel Tap

Lay down on your back with your knees in a bent position and your heels near your bottom.

Lift your shoulders slightly away from the floor, engage abs and reach one hand down by your side to tap your heel.

Repeat and alternate.

Aim to keep shoulders off the floor, and don't hold your breath!

Stretch & Relax

Seated tree pose (Yoga - 'Vrkasana').

Sit down with one leg stretched straight out in front of you with your foot flexed and place your other foot at your inner thigh.

Sit up tall with a long, straight spine and neutral neck, breathe in and raise the hands in the air.

Lean forward over the extended leg with your hands towards your foot.

Either hold onto the foot and draw yourself further forward or again use a small towel to achieve this.

Reverse and repeat on the other side.

Hold for at least 1 minute and move with the breath by sinking deeper into the stretch with each exhalation.

Instructional videos available at **www.superfoodist.com**

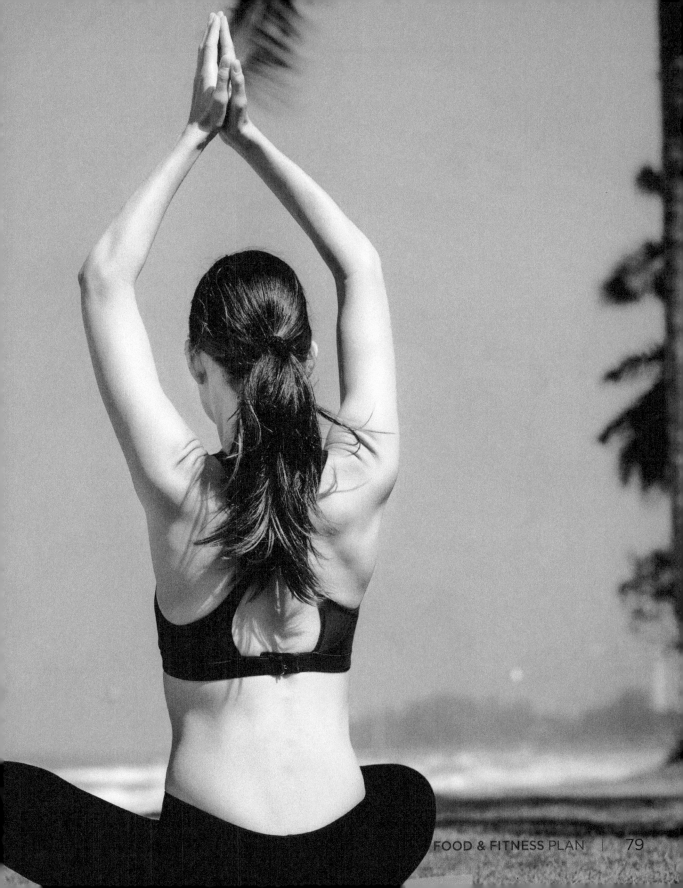

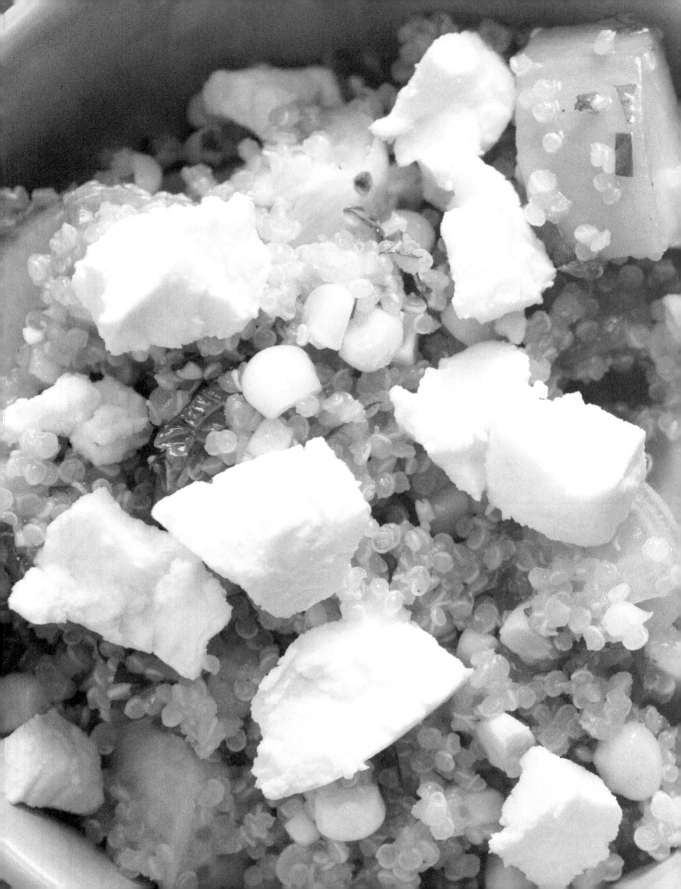

Weeks
6&8

Rev Up

Breakfast

Blueberry, Rhubarb and Apple Porridge

Add 3 tablespoons of antioxidant rich blueberries, stewed rhubarb or stewed apples to a small bowl of porridge.

The oats help keep blood sugar levels stable and assist with cravings whilst the fruit helps to keep your immune system strong.

This breakfast is both calming and stimulating to the digestive tract.

OR

Raspberry Smoothie

Blend 250mls of unsweetened rice or almond milk with a cup of fresh or frozen raspberries.

Add 1 scoop of Plant Based Protein like Sunwarrior Natural, Vanilla or Chocolate.

Then add 5 or 6 almonds to promote satiety.

OR

Small Mixed Berry Bowl

Have 1 cup of fresh or frozen berries with a dollop of organic natural yogurt or coconut yogurt.

Top with 5 or 6 almonds.

The berries are phytonutrient dense superfood option that help keep your immune system strong whilst the nuts provide some protein to help keep you full and focused.

AND

Tea, Coffee or Herbal Tea

1 Cup of coffee, tea or herbal tea of choice to help with fullness and hydration.

The caffeine in the coffee or tea has fat burning qualities but choose a calming herbal variety if anxiety is an issue.

Sweeten with a little honey, stevia or xylitol.

Do not use sugar or artificial sweeteners.

Before Breakfast

Grapefruit Blast

One glass or cup of warm filtered water with the juice of half a grapefruit and a little cinnamon to kick start digestion and fat metabolism.

This morning combination also regulates blood sugar levels thereby helping to reduce cravings.

Mid Morning

Dates, Nut and Seed Mix

Have 3 or 4 dates to help with regularity - if you're constipated it's harder to lose weight.

Also have 3 teaspoons of mixed nuts and seeds as the protein content will keep you satisfied.

OR

Almonds and Apple

1 Apple with 8 - 10 almonds is the prefect snack to promote fullness. The pectin in the apple combines perfectly with the protein in the nuts to ensure satiety.

OR

Herbal Tea

1 Cup of herbal tea
Spearmint or Peppermint both aid digestive function.

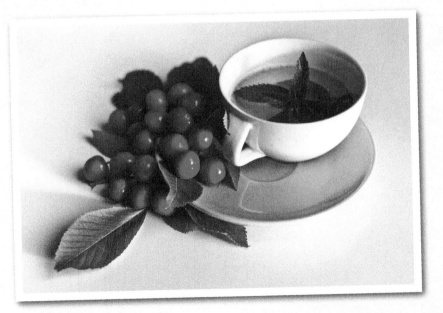

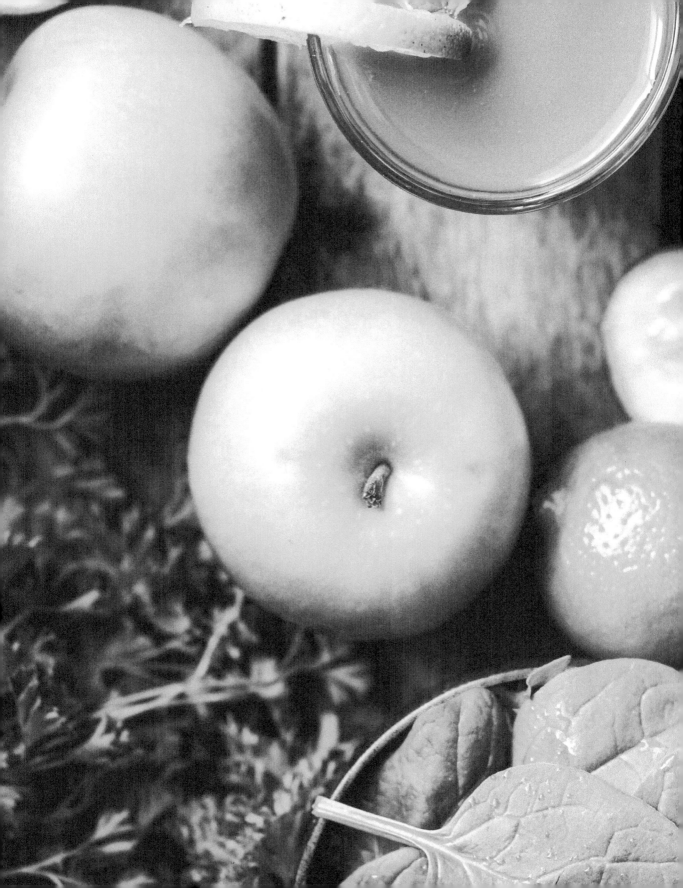

Before Lunch & Dinner

Spirulina Super Green Boost

6 Spirulina or Super Green tablets can be taken as they help with feelings of fullness and with controlling portion size.

They also help to alkalise, detox and cleanse.

Lunch

Cayenne Tuna Green Vegetables

Add half a cup of steamed mixed green vegetables and a few slices of red pepper to a small tin of tuna.

Season with chilli cayenne and shallots.

Serve with half a cup of brown rice.

OR

Avocado and Tomato Cream Cheese Corn Crackers

Top 2 corn crackers with a light spread of avocado, tomato and cream cheese.

These crackers are high in protein and healthy omegas to help with satiety.

Add black pepper and turmeric to stimulate digestion.

OR

Beans and Salad Open Sandwich

Use 1 piece of wholegrain crispbread such as Ryvita for the base.

Add a generous portion of lentils, chick peas or red kidney beans and salad leaves to make an open sandwich.

Season with black pepper, sea salt and chilli.

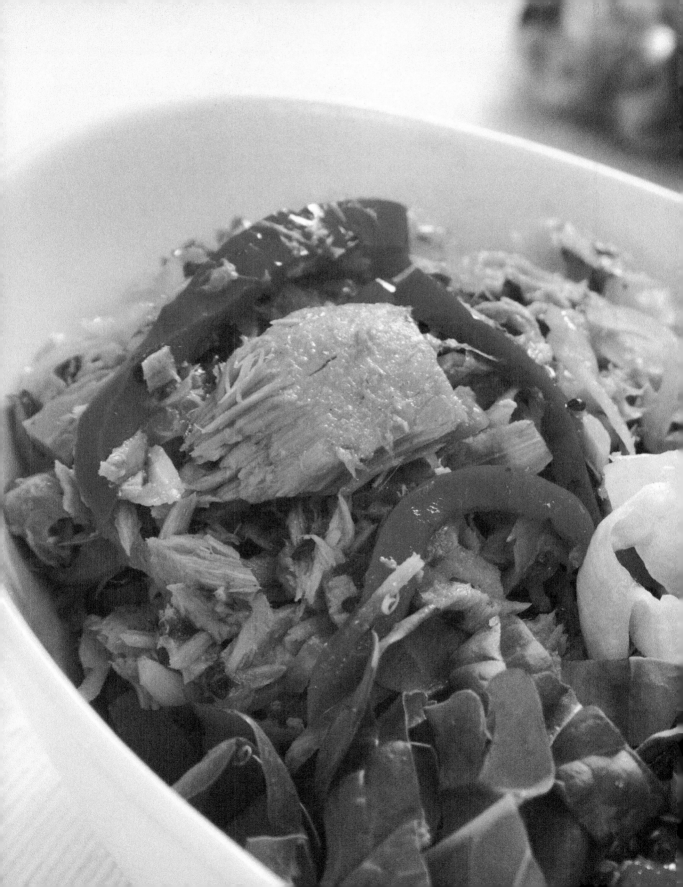

Mid Afternoon

Boiled Egg with Pepper

Organic or Free Range Boiled Egg with black pepper.
A protein source with a thermogenic spice to help reduce cravings.

OR

Avocado Sticks

Mash half an avocado and serve with 4 or 5 small carrot or celery sticks.
Add cayenne to spice things up.

AND

Spearmint or Peppermint Tea

Both of these teas are digestive tonics.

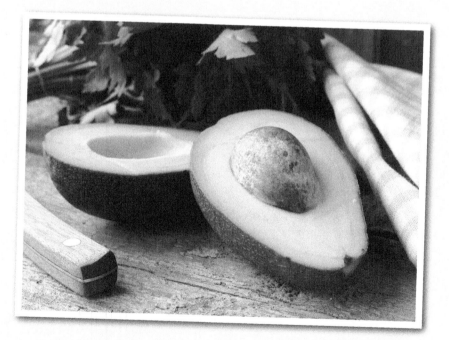

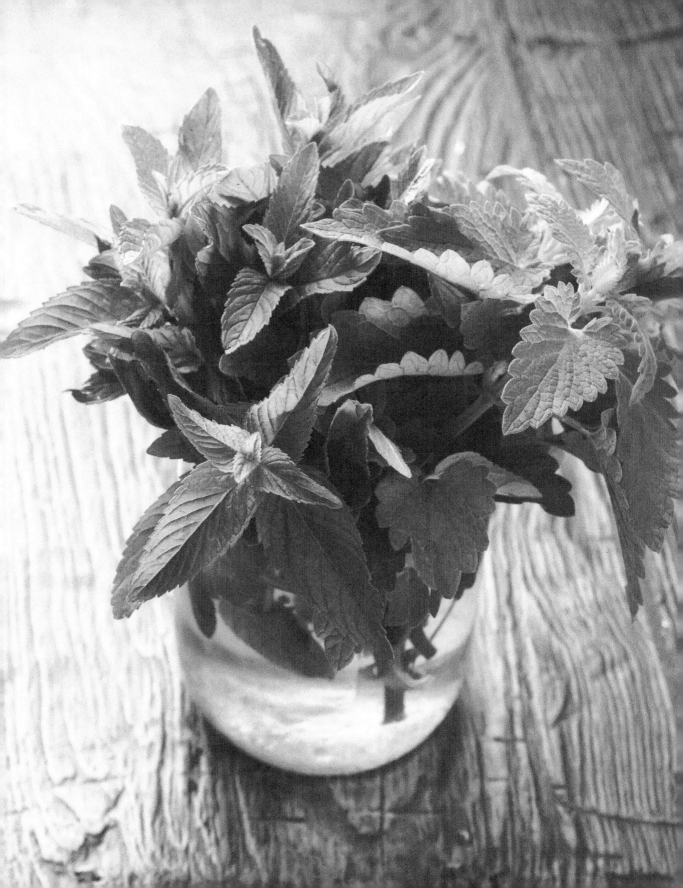

Dinner

Vegetable Lentil Soup

Add a cup of pre-cooked lentils or mixed beans and 2 cups of mixed vegetables to 300/400mls of water.

Simmer slowly and add turmeric, chilli and ginger.

Have with 1 small slice of wholegrain toast.

Soups are a great choice when on a weight management campaign - they are hydrating, filling and easy on the digestive system.

OR

Mediterranean Chilli Roast Vegetables

2 cups of any vegetables such as red onion, courgette, peppers and tomatoes.

Bake for 20 minutes in a small lasagne dish with a drizzle of cold pressed olive oil and garlic, herb and chilli seasoning.

You could also add half a cup of lentils or chick peas to increase the protein content of this meal.

OR

Blueberry Smoothie

Blend 250mls of unsweetened rice or almond milk with a cup of fresh or frozen blueberries.

Add 1 scoop of Plant Based Protein Powder like Sunwarrior - Natural, Vanilla or Chocolate - and 5 or 6 almonds to promote satiety.

AND

Spearmint, Peppermint, Fennel or Dandelion Tea

All of these teas are digestive and liver tonics.

After Dinner:

Stewed Pears

Stew one pear in a little filtered water and add some sultanas or raisins.

Top with a little cinnamon, chilli or cayenne to regulate blood sugar and boost fat burning.

Before Bed

Calming Sleepy Tea

1 Cup of calming herbal tea

Choose either chamomile, lemon balm or valerian to nourish the nervous system.

Exercises for
Weeks 6&8

Warm Up
1 Minute Cardio - Jumping Jacks

Begin by simply stepping from side to side raising your hands and arms up above you as you do so.

Then move your arms down again in coordination with your steps.
To increase the intensity start to move the legs out whilst raising the arms at the same time.

Increase speed to intensify further.

HIIT Circuit Weeks 6&8

Do each exercise in the circuit for 30 seconds intensely and then slowly for 30 seconds.

Each individual exercise within the circuit should be done for 1 minute.

Beginner - complete once or twice
Intermediate - complete two or three times
Advanced - complete three or four times

Reverse Lunge with Toe (High Kick) Touch

Start in a standing position with your hands on your hips.

Take a step back and lower the back knee towards the floor in a lunge position.

Then push off from that back foot to bring that leg forward in front of your body with the knee bent to a 90 degree angle - repeat x5.

Repeat on other side.

Bridge with Knee Raise

Lie flat on your back with your knees in a bent knee position with your heels towards your bottom.

Your lower back should be pressed into the floor with a small natural arch at the lower spine to activate the core.

Raise the hips away from the ground to a bridge pose and at the same time lift one knee towards your chest while squeezing the glutes.

Return to the floor and repeat on the other side.

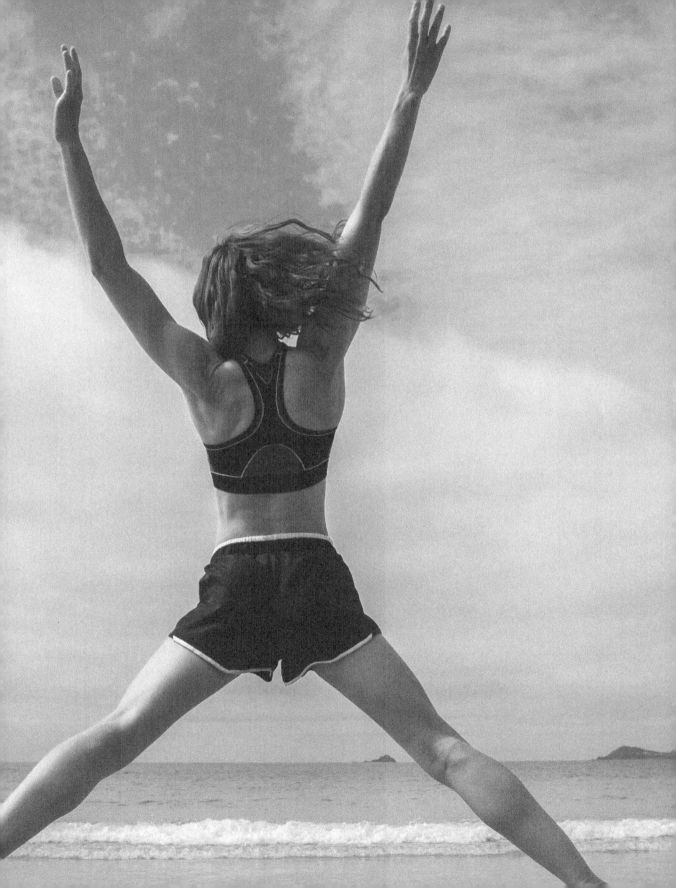

Roll Down with Push Up

Begin in a standing position with your core engaged.

Start to slide your hands down toward the ground bending your knees until the hands are flat on the floor.

Then walk the hands forward until you are in a high Plank position.

Perform either a full or half push up before walking the hands back and rolling back up to a standing position.

Repeat for allotted time.

Abs - Crunch

Lay down with your knees bent.

Your feet should hover above ground about 2 cms or 1 inch.

Pull your knees to your chest keeping the calves resting against your hamstrings as you raise your shoulders from the floor to meet your knees.

Make sure you keep your neck neutral and don't bend it forward.

Stretch & Relax

Lunge pose into Pyramid pose (Yoga - 'Parsvottonasana').

Start with the right foot placed between your hands on the floor.

Stretch out your left leg behind you in a lunge or runner's position, stretching out your hip flexor (thigh) and glute.

Hold here for 15 - 20 seconds then straighten the front right leg to form a triangle or pyramid shape with your legs.

Make sure to keep this front leg in a straight position.

Reach you hands down towards the right foot - either have your hands flat on the floor or hold onto your ankle or leg if less flexible.

Repeat on the other side.

Instructional videos available at **www.superfoodist.com**

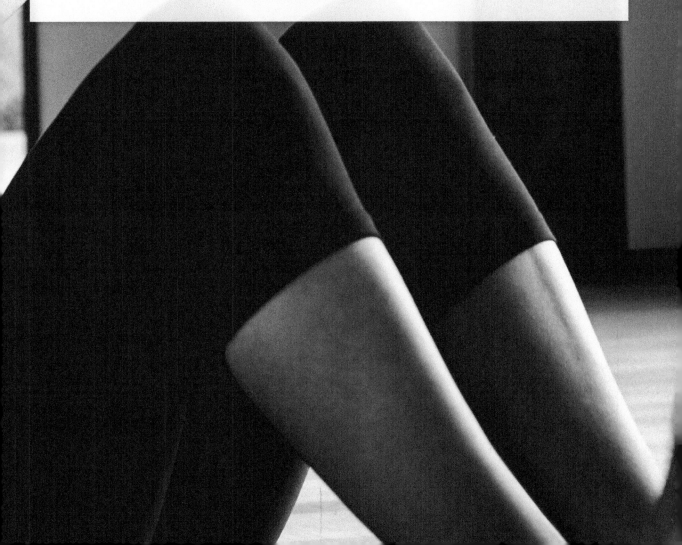

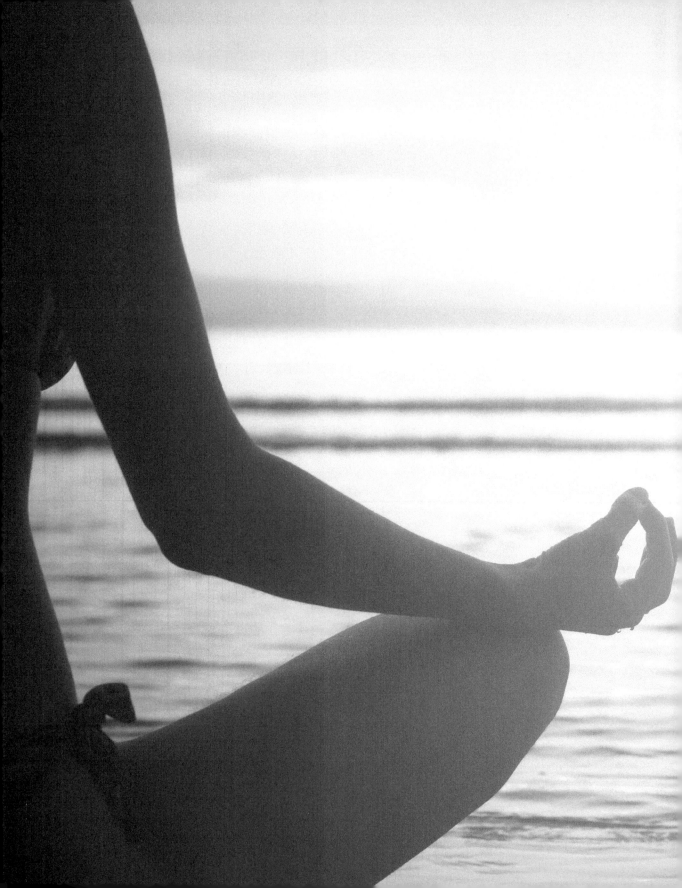

intro Weeks 9 to 12

Congratulations on making it to the final four weeks of your health and fitness transformation!

The final four weeks of your Anti Ageing Food and Fitness Plan really help you to shed those unwanted pounds and to increase your fitness level. You should also see an improvement in mood, energy and fitness.

This part of the plan has been formulated using the latest scientific research to promote weight loss and fat burning - again it is high in protein, is nutrient dense, is low in calories and is designed to keep the glycaemic load of meals and snacks down.

There are benefits to the digestive, nervous and circulatory systems and you can expect hair, skin and nail health to improve as well.

These four weeks follow the principles of intermittent fasting whereby fewer calories are consumed over a two day period in the week. The two days when you consume fewer calories can be any that you choose in the week - they do not need to be two consecutive days.

During the final four weeks of the plan you are encouraged to do some moderate exercise five times per week in order to achieve optimal results. High intensity interval training exercises have been chosen as these will get you the best fitness results in the shortest amount of time.

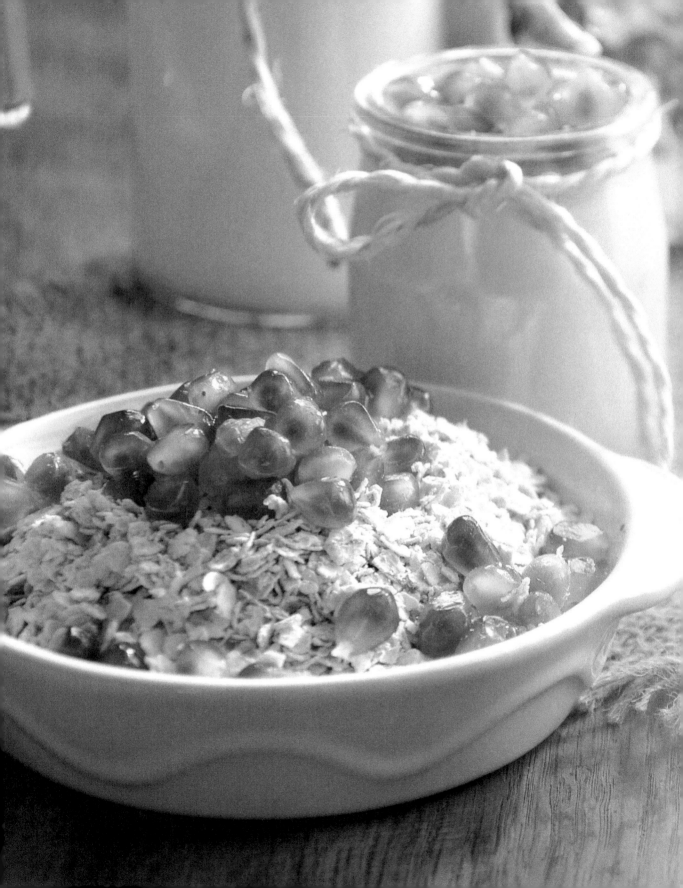

Weeks
9to12

5 Days a Week

Tone Up

Before Breakfast
Grapefruit or Lemon Kick Starter
One glass or cup of warm water with the juice of half a grapefruit or lemon in order to stimulate digestion and to help with fat metabolism.

Add a dash of cinnamon to stabilise blood sugar levels and reduce cravings whilst promoting a calm mood.

Breakfast

Spicy Baked Beans

Half a tin of organic low salt baked beans on 2 slices of wholemeal or rye toast.

Add some chilli or tabasco to the beans which act as thermogenic agents to speed up the metabolism and stimulate the digestion. High in protein with some carbs for energy.

OR

Nut, Apple and Fruit Breakfast Bowl

Cut up 1 small apples and add a quarter of a cup of raw unsalted mixed nuts.

A few pieces of dried fruit such as dates, raisins or sultanas can also be added to help increase energy production.

Mix together in a bowl with a glass of unsweetened rice or almond milk - more energy and fibre from the dates and satiety from the nuts.

A handful of oats can be added to the mix to help promote fullness even more.

OR

Super Berry Smoothie

Blend 250mls of unsweetened rice or almond milk together with 1 small banana and half a cup of fresh or frozen berries.

1 Scoop of Plant Based Protein such as Sunwarrior - Natural, Vanilla or Chocolate can be added to increase satiety as can a handful of almonds.

AND

Coffee / Tea or Herbal Tea

1 Cup of coffee, tea or herbal tea of choice sweetened with a little honey, stevia or xylitol - no added sugar or artificial sweeteners are to be used.

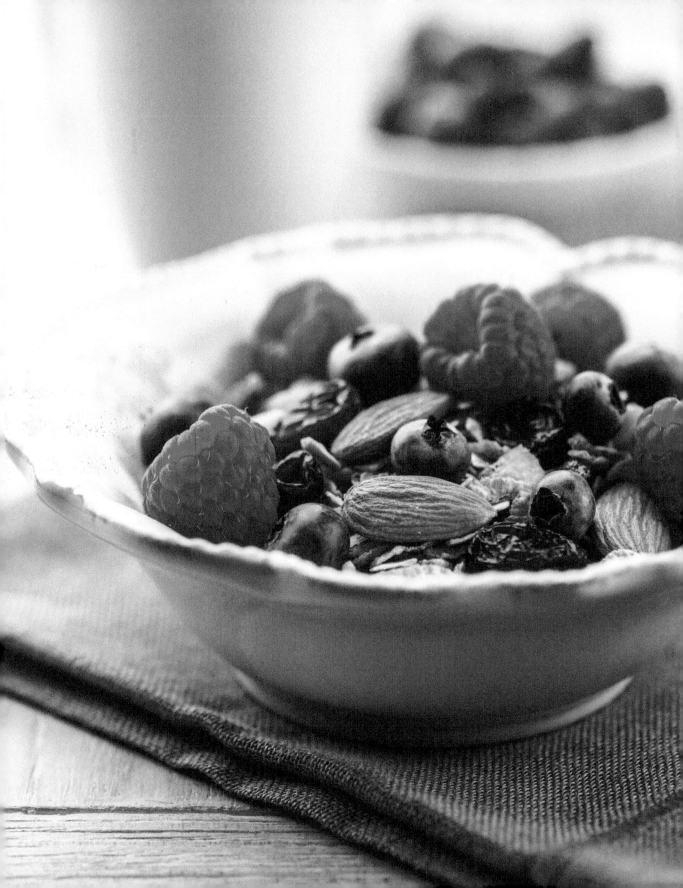

Mid Morning

Seasonal Fruit with Almonds and Seeds

Have a small bowl of seasonal fruit topped with 5 or 6 almonds.

This can be served with a few teaspoons of coconut yogurt.

The fruit and nuts are nutrient dense and help with both cognitive and immune function with the nuts providing protein to help with fullness.

OR

Apple and Pecan Snack

1 Apple with 6 - 8 pecans.

This snack combines pectin and protein to keep mid morning cravings at bay.

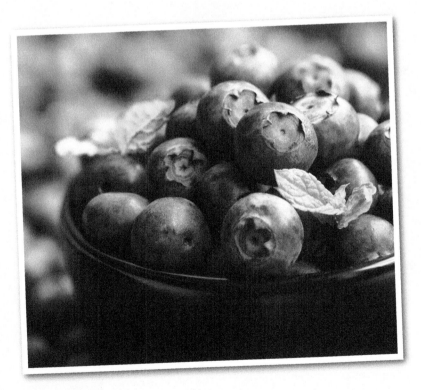

Before Lunch & Dinner

Spirulina Super Green Boost

Before lunch or dinner have up to 6 Spirulina or Super Greens tablets to assist with detox, cleansing and weight control.

Lunch

Spicy Avocado Omelette

2 or 3 Organic or free range egg omelette or scrambled eggs with no added milk or cheese.
Serve with half an avocado.
Season with chilli, cayenne or black pepper.

OR

Vegetarian Sausages with Asparagus, Broccoli, Tomato and Beans

Lightly fry 2 Vegetarian Sausages in cold pressed olive oil.
Steam a cup sized portion of asparagus, broccoli and green beans together with 3 or 4 cherry tomatoes.
Add olive oil, balsamic vinegar and fresh cracked black pepper.

OR

Rice Salad with Pine Nuts and Cashews

Add half a cup of any combination of steamed green vegetables to half a cup of brown rice.
Top with a handful of pine nuts and cashews to boost the protein content of this meal option.

Mid Afternoon

Banana Delight

2 or 3 Dates or a glass of organic prune juice with 1 banana.
If you're constipated it's harder to lose weight - the banana provides fibre and energy that will boost you both physically and mentally.
Have two teaspoons of mixed nuts and seeds if you want a higher protein content.

AND

Peppermint or Spearmint Tea

A cup of peppermint or spearmint tea with a little added honey to both calm and stimulate digestion.

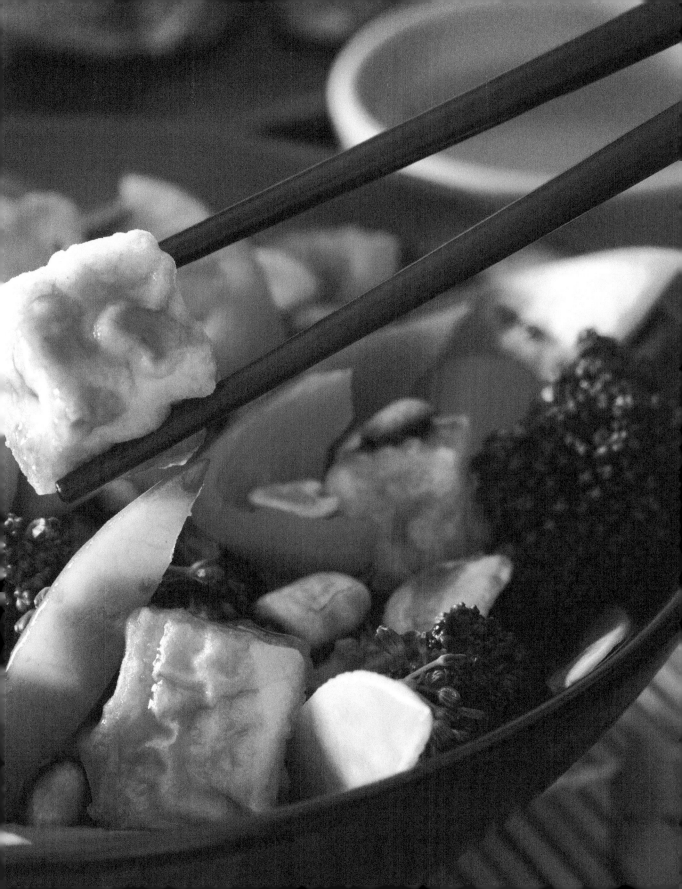

Dinner

Bunless Burger with Mustard and Pine Nuts

Lightly fry a vegetarian burger option in cold pressed olive oil and serve with a cupful of leafy salad greens or steamed greens and a teaspoon or two of pine nuts.
Top with a mustard and chilli dressing.

OR

Grilled Tofu, Salmon or Tuna with Green Leaves

Grill a small piece of one the protein sources above and serve with green leaves or steamed greens.
Dress with balsamic vinegar, black pepper and sea salt.

OR

Vegetable stir fry with Cashews

Lightly stir fry in cold pressed olive oil a vegetable medley of your choice.
Add 10 or 11 raw cashews and make sure you add spices to taste to stimulate digestive juices and speed up metabolism.
Serve with 3/4 cup of brown rice.
Use soy sauce, ginger, chilli and garlic.

AND

Dandelion Tea

One cup of dandelion tea - the bitter qualities of this tea aid liver and gall bladder function making it good for weight loss, fluid retention, bloating and skin conditions.

After Dinner

Stewed Cinnamon Apples or Pears with Almonds
Slowly stew 1 apple or 1 pear and serve with a topping of cinnamon and half a teaspoon of almond slivers.

Before Bed

Sleepy Tea
1 Cup of herbal tea such as chamomile, lemon balm or valerian

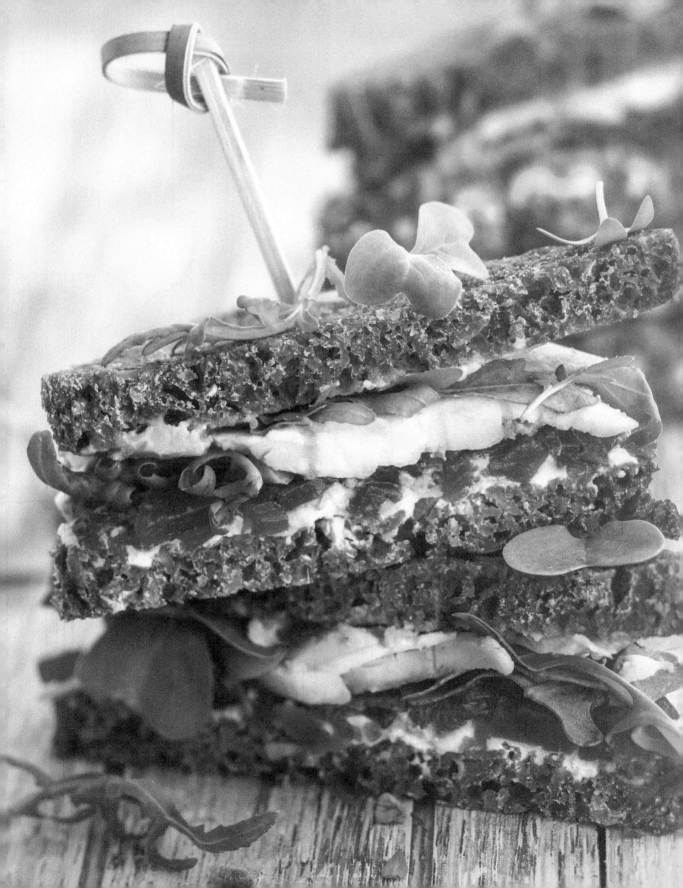

Weeks
9 to 12

2 Days a Week

Tone up
Turbo Charge

Before Breakfast
Lemon Grapefruit Blast

One glass or cup of warm filtered water with the juices of half a lemon and a quarter of a grapefruit and a little cinnamon and honey to kick start digestion and fat metabolism.

This blast also regulates blood sugar levels to help stop cravings.

Breakfast
Raspberry Smoothie

Blend 250mls of unsweetened rice, oat, coconut or almond milk with 1 small banana chopped, half a cup of raspberries and a handful of spinach or kale.

OR

Berry Bowl

1 Cup of mixed berries - fresh or frozen - with a dollop of unsweetened organic yogurt.

The berries are a nutrient dense superfood that help keep your immune system strong whilst the yogurt provides protein to help keep you full and focused.

OR

Chickpea Breakfast Soup

Blend half a can of organic chickpeas with a quarter of a teaspoon of tumeric, ginger and black pepper.

Add some sea salt or rock salt and 200mls of filtered water.

Soup is a great breakfast option particularly if it's protein based. This soup is filling and the spices have thermogenic properties.

AND

Green Tea

1 Cup of green or Matcha tea to help burn and metabolise fat.

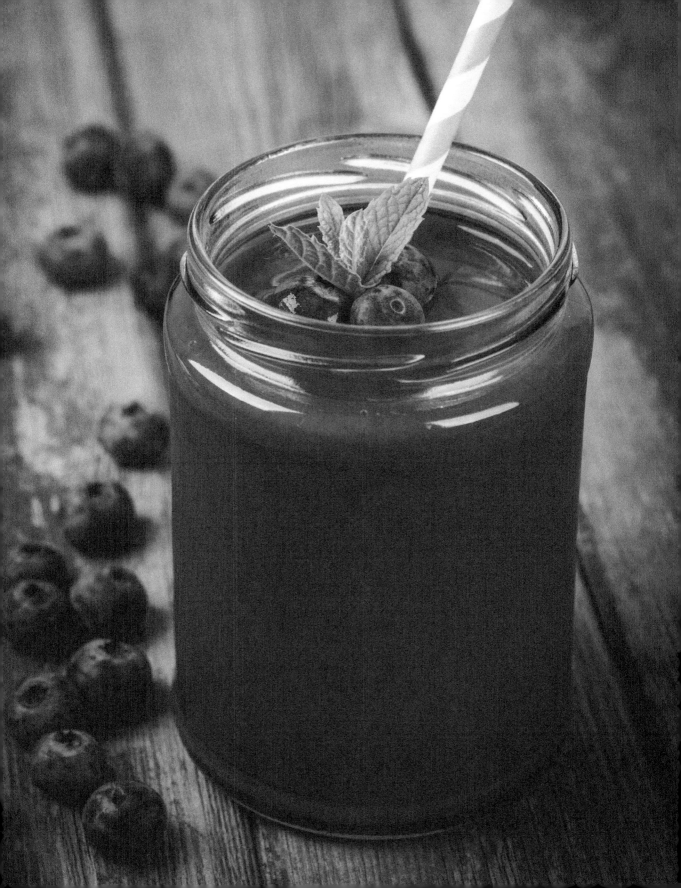

Mid Morning

Prune, Nut and Seed Snack

3 or 4 Prunes or a glass of organic prune juice if you prefer.
Remember if you're constipated it's harder to lose weight.
Have 3 teaspoons of mixed nuts and seeds - for protein to help keep you satisfied.

OR

Apple and Almonds

1 Apple with 8 - 10 almonds will keep your sugar cravings at bay.

AND

Spearmint or Peppermint Tea

1 Cup of herbal tea to keep digestive function at an optimal level.

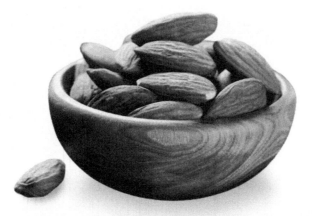

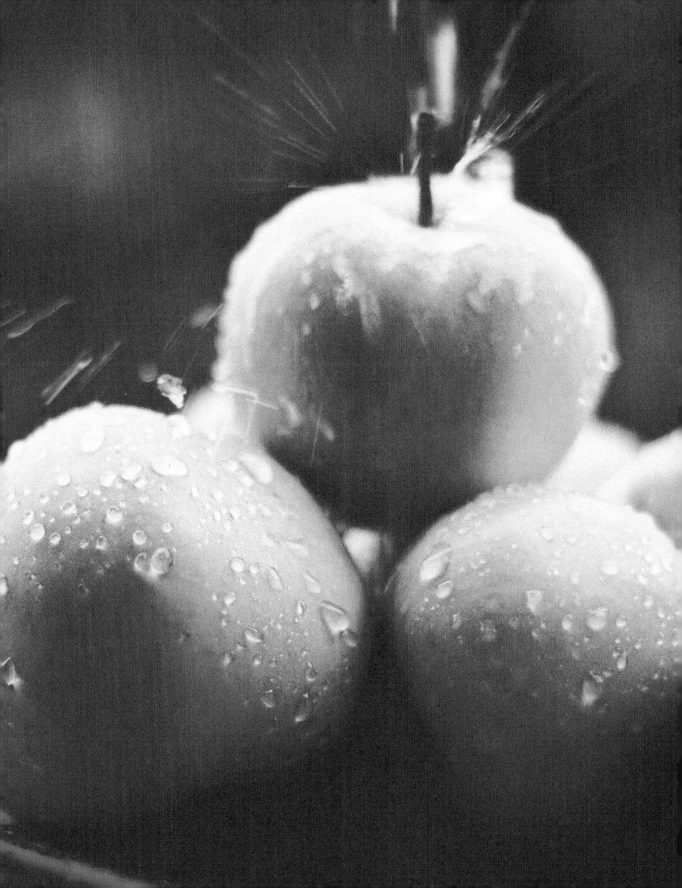

Before Lunch & Dinner

Spirulina Super Green Boost

Before lunch and dinner up to 6 Spirulina or Super Green tablets can be taken as they help with feelings of fullness and with controlling portion size.

They also help to alkalise, cleanse and detox the system.

Lunch

Green Smoothie

Blend 1 pear, 2 celery stalks, 1 inch slice of ginger, 2 cups of chard, 1/2 an avocado and 1 teaspoon of chia seeds with 200mls of coconut water. Add a pinch of chilli or cayenne for a thermogenic boost.

OR

Avocado and Tomato Crackers

2 Wholegrain crackers topped with avocado thinly spread and tomato. Sprinkle on some sea salt and black pepper to taste.

This light lunch is high in protein and healthy omegas to help with satiety.

OR

Open Salad Sandwich

Use a generous handful of lentils, chick peas or red kidney beans with salad leaves to make an open sandwich.

Use 1 piece of wholegrain crispbread as the base.

Season with black pepper.

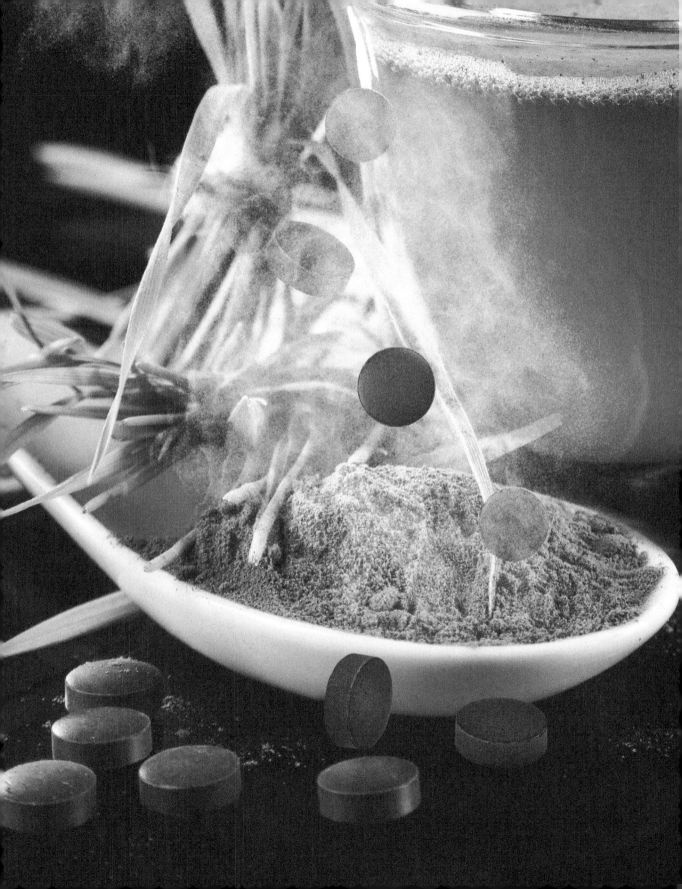

Mid Afternoon

Peppered Egg

1 Boiled organic or free range egg with black pepper. Quick protein with a thermogenic spice to help reduce cravings.

OR

Mashed Avocado and Carrot or Celery Sticks

Half an avocado mashed served with 4 or 5 small carrots or celery sticks.

AND

Dandelion Tea or Coffee

1 Cup of dandelion tea to stimulate the liver and gall bladder and to assist with the digestive process.

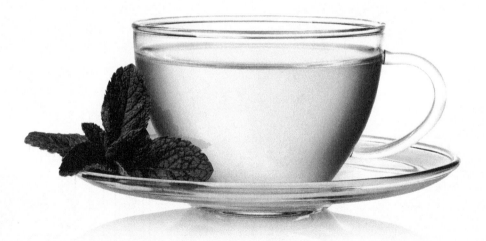

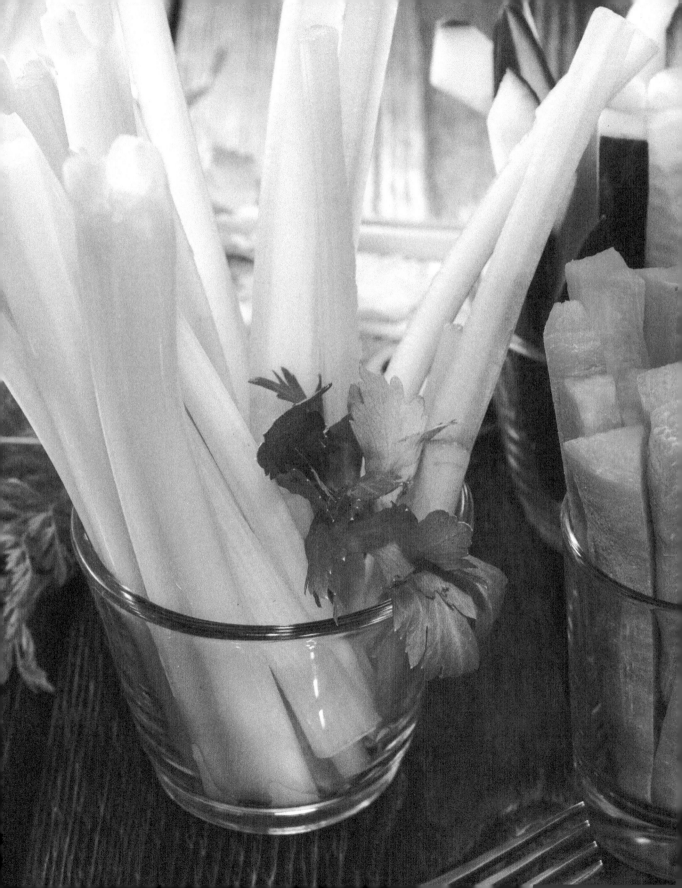

Dinner

Lentil Ginger and Chilli Soup

Add a cup of lentils or beans plus 2 cups of green vegetables to 300/400mls of water.

Simmer slowly and add turmeric, chilli and ginger.

This is easy to digest and thermogenic spices help speed up fat loss.

OR

Chilli Roast Mediterranean Chick Pea Vegetables

Any combination of 2 cups of vegetables such as red onion, courgette, peppers and tomatoes with a garlic, herb and chilli seasoning.

Add half a cup of chick peas.

Bake in a small lasagne dish with a drizzle of cold pressed olive oil.

OR

Berry and Chia Immune Booster

Blend 2 cups of mixed berries, half a banana, 1 teaspoon of chia seeds, 1 teaspoon of linseeds, 1 teaspoon of pumpkin or sunflower seeds, 7 almonds and 200mls of water or coconut water.

The nuts and seeds combined with the berries make this the perfect phytonutrient rich light dinner that won't leave you feeling hungry.

AND

Green Tea
1 Cup of green tea.

Before Bed

Sleepy Tea
1 Cup of herbal tea such as chamomile, lemon balm or valerian.

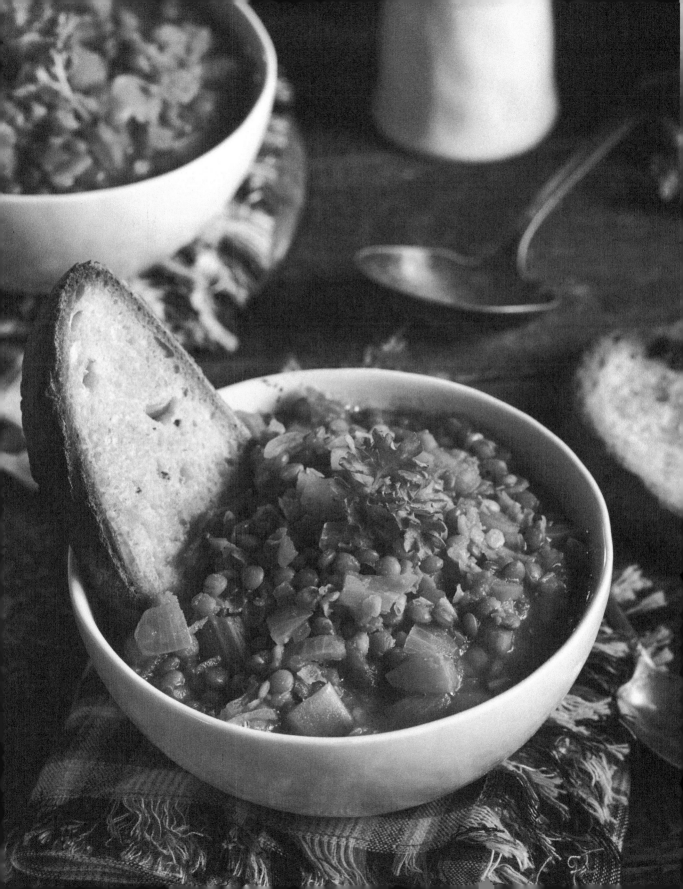

Exercises for
Weeks 9&11

Warm Up
1 Minute Cardio - Jump Ups

Start by having the feet fairly close together about shoulder width apart beginning with little jumps in the air.

After 10 seconds begin to jump up a bit higher from a squat position and start to also raise both knees in the air in front of you at the same time.

Try to make sure you land softly on your toes not your heels or on flat feet. Increase intensity by jumping higher and faster bringing your knees up high. Try to do for 1 minute.

HIIT Circuit Weeks 9&11

Do each exercise in the circuit for 40 seconds intensely and then slowly for 20 seconds.

Each individual exercise within the circuit should be done for 1 minute.

Beginner - complete once or twice
Intermediate - complete two or three times
Advanced - complete three or four times

Punches

Holding your hands up in front of your face punch forward in an alternating action.

Perform 10 forward punches and 10 hooks from side to side then 10 uppercuts.

Lunge Jumps

Start in a lunge position, then simply jump up in the air landing with your feet in the opposite positions.

Jump higher in the air to increase intensity.

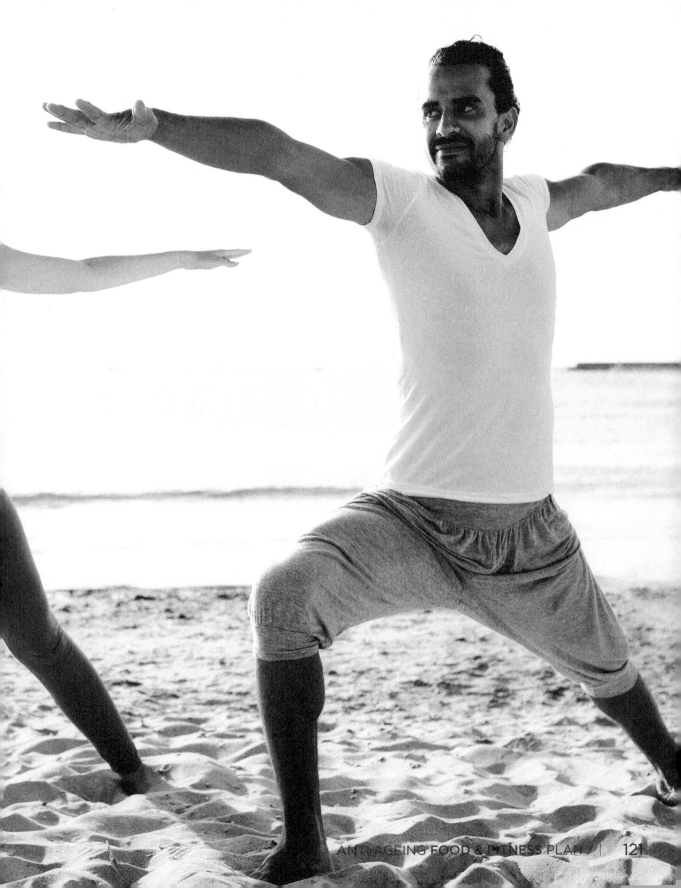

Superwoman

Start by lying down in a face down position.
Stretch out your arms straight in front and stretch your legs straight behind.
Engage your core by drawing the belly button to the spine.
Take a breath in and as you exhale lift both the arms and legs (from the hips if possible) at the same time.
Hold for a count of 2 and release back to your starting position. Repeat.

Abs Bicycle

Lay on your back with your lower legs in a tabletop position.
Slightly raise shoulders from floor with hands behind head.
Alternate moving your elbow towards your opposite knee in a fast motion, with your legs moving in a cycling action.

Stretch & Relax

Half Pigeon Pose (Yoga - 'Eka Pada Rajakapotasana').
Start on all fours.
Bring your left knee forward and place it just behind and slightly to the left of your left wrist.
Place the lower leg at either a right angle (only for the most flexible) but probably at around 45 degrees toward the right inner thigh.
Stretch your right leg out behind you and fold your torso forwards and over your bent left leg - make sure to keep your hips balanced and don't over rotate.
Hold for 1 min and repeat on the other side.

Instructional videos available at **www.superfoodist.com**

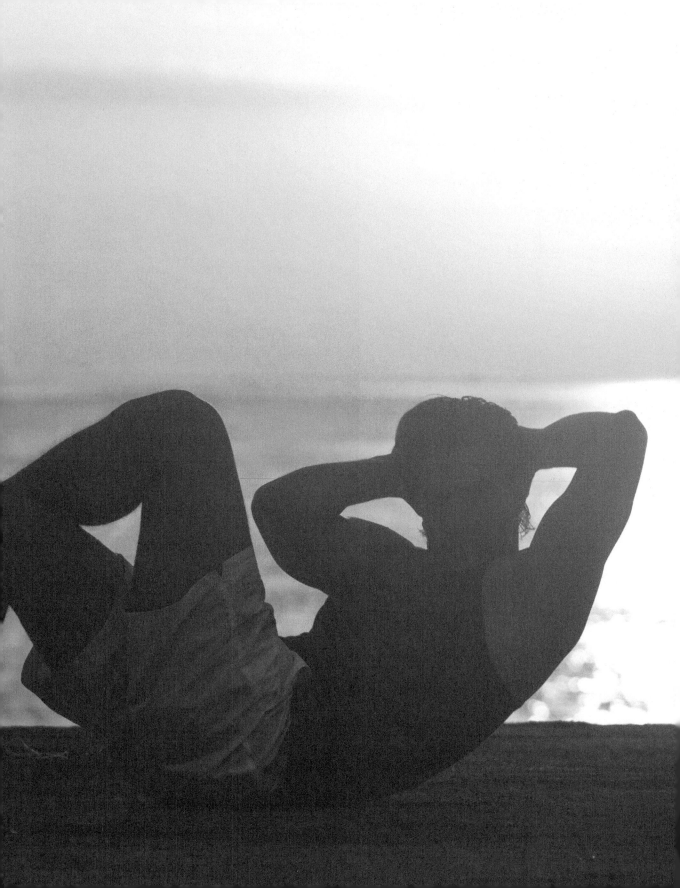

Exercises for
Weeks 10&12

Warm Up
1 Minute Cardio - Star Cross Overs

Stand with your legs more than shoulder width apart with your arms out to the side and parallel to the ground.

Take your right hand and reach down toward your left foot bending forward as well.

Return to the star position and repeat on the other side.

To increase the intensity increase the speed of motion, windmilling from side to side.

HIIT Circuit Weeks 10&12

Do each exercise in the circuit for 40 seconds intensely and then slowly for 20 seconds.

Each individual exercise within the circuit should be done for 1 minute.

Beginner - complete once or twice
Intermediate - complete two or three times
Advanced - complete three or four times

Multi-Planar Jump Backs

The basic position here is a high Plank.

Begin by jumping the feet together towards the elbows to a crouch position then jump back to one side, i.e. about a 45 degree angle.

Keep jumping back and forth changing the direction to the other side.

Keep repeating all three positions, alternating sides.

To decrease the intensity you can walk the legs to/from the position so as to slow down the movement.

Push Ups

Beginners: Start on your knees with your feet away from the floor.
Keep your hips in line with your shoulders and knees.
Keep the hips level and lower the torso toward the ground and push
back to your starting position.

Advanced: Raise your knees from the floor and perform
the movement on your toes.
Move your hands further apart to work the
chest more and move them closer to
work the triceps.

Prisoner Squat & Kick

Holding your hands behind your head go down to a squat.

As you stand back up kick one leg forward on the way up. Repeat alternating legs.

Squat deeper to increase intensity.

Abs - Leg Raise

Lay on your back with your legs straight up in the air with your soles facing the ceiling.

Raise the feet higher and lift the lower back from the floor, which exercises the lower abdominals.

Lower and repeat.

Stretch & Relax

Half King Fish Pose (Yoga - 'Ardha Matsyendrasana').

This is a half spinal twist pose and a full body stretch.

Start by sitting up straight, with your legs out in front.

Take the left foot and place it over the right knee.

Bring the right elbow around and place it on the outside of the left knee.

Place the left hand behind you - applying a little pressure on the left knee with the elbow.

Look over your left shoulder whilst feeling the full stretch.

To progress the pose bend the right leg round so that your foot is near your left glute.

Hold for at least 1 minute.

Reverse and repeat on the opposite side.

Instructional videos available at **www.superfoodist.com**

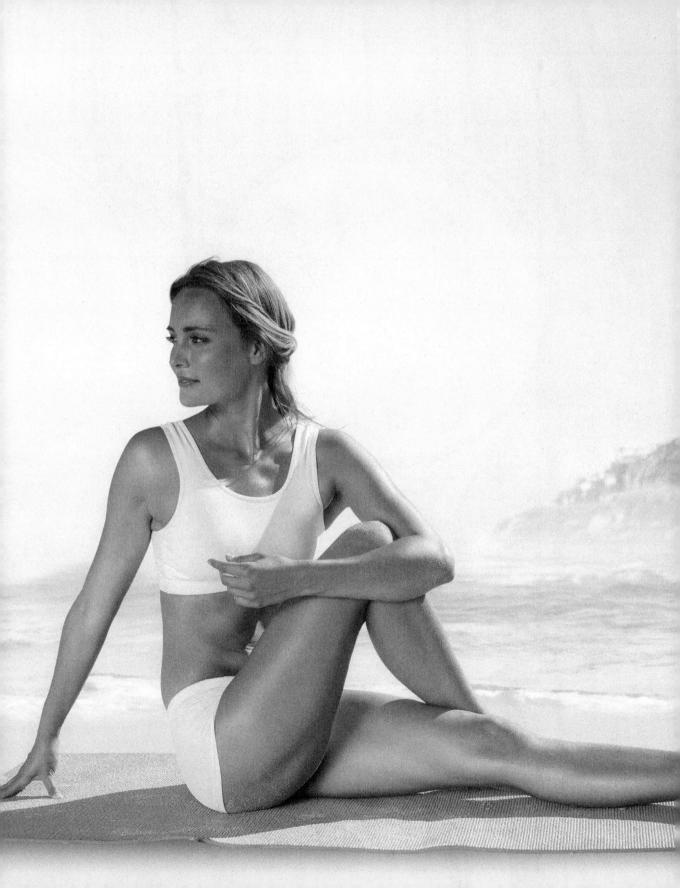

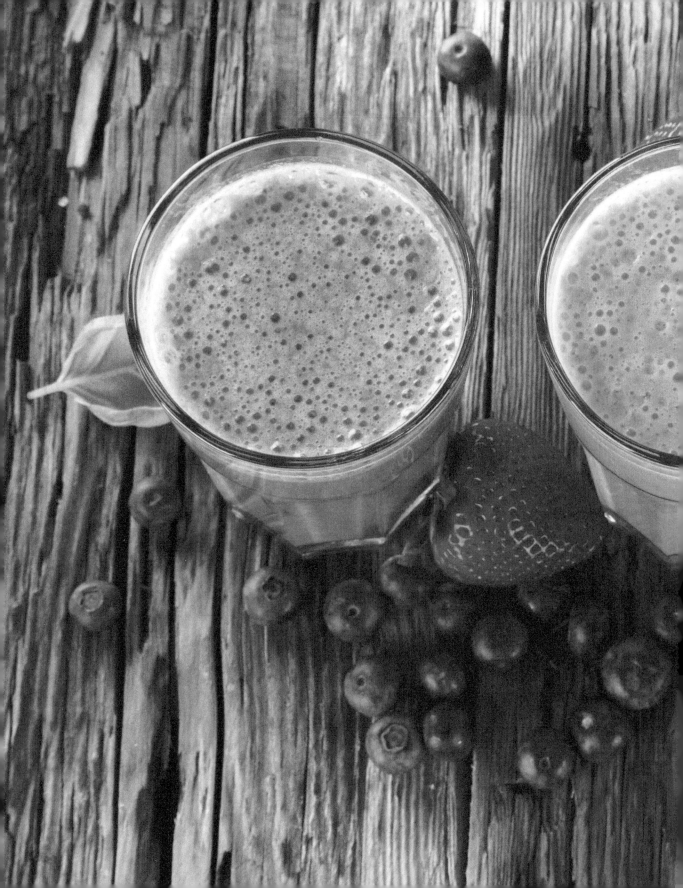

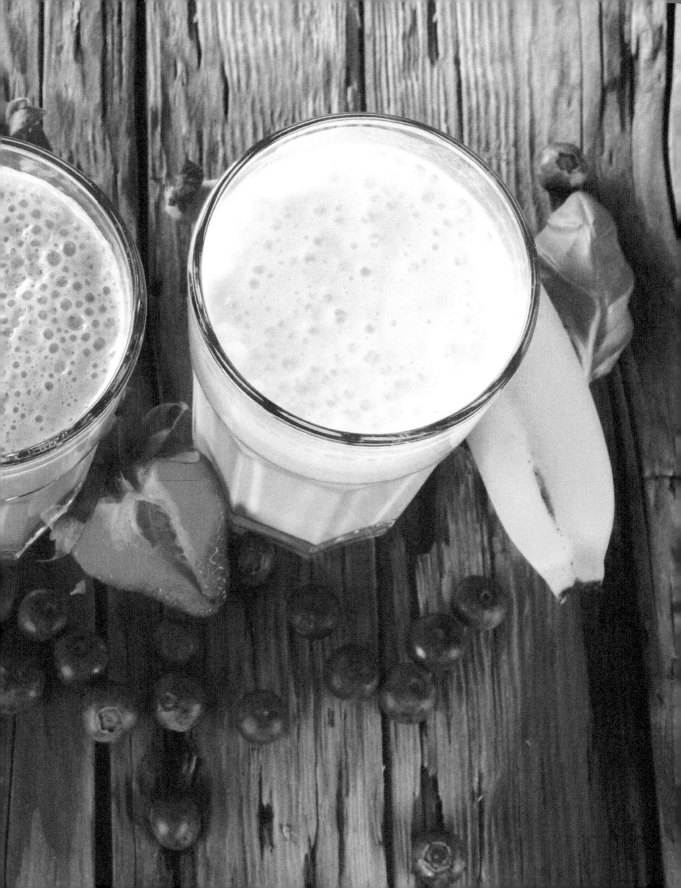

Go Figa
The Superfood Fig Powder

Go Figa is a nutrient dense superfood that has been designed to help boost immunity, regulate blood sugar levels, help with regularity and promote satiety.

This formula includes antioxidant rich fig powder combined with berries, chia seeds, cinnamon and glucomannan.

The combination of ingredients has been selected to assist natural cleansing and detox processes whilst delivering a general tune up to all body systems.

Go Figa is packed full of phytonutrients which assist with digestive function and energy production.

Our Super Blend powder is designed to assist with:
~ Digestive function
~ Regularity
~ Satiety

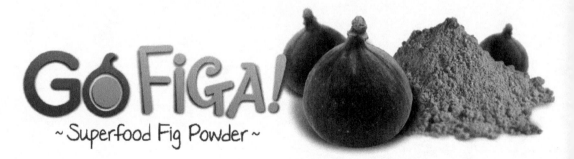

Go Figa is available from **www.thesuperfoodist.com**

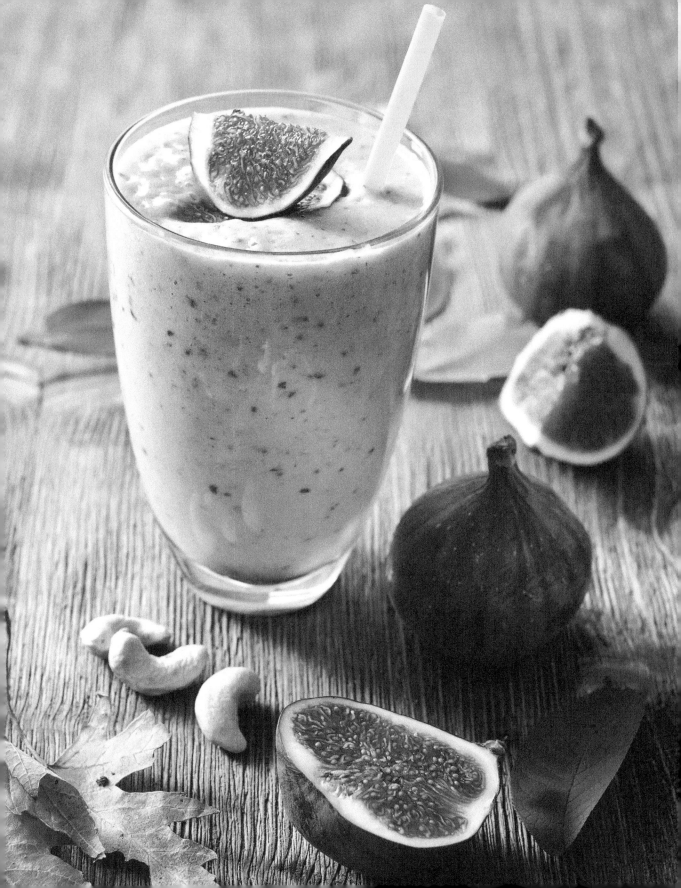

Go Boost
The Superfood Fruit Powder

Go Boost is an organic superfood blend that will assist with energy production and boost immunity.

This antioxidant powerhouse includes the Superberries Goji and Acai together with Vitamin C rich Lucuma and Baobab.
It also contains Banana and Maca powder for a natural energy lift.

Go Boost is a good source of potassium and zinc and also contains iron which can reduce tiredness and fatigue.

Take once or twice daily in a little water prior to exercise or you can add it to one of your daily juices or smoothies.
Go Boost can be taken post exercise to assist with toning and lean muscle mass.

It can also be taken in a little water or juice mid morning or mid afternoon to provide a natural energy lift.

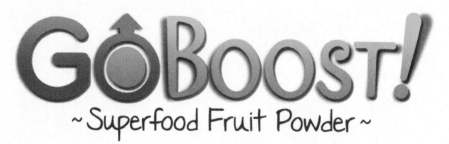

Go Boost is available from **www.thesuperfoodist.com**

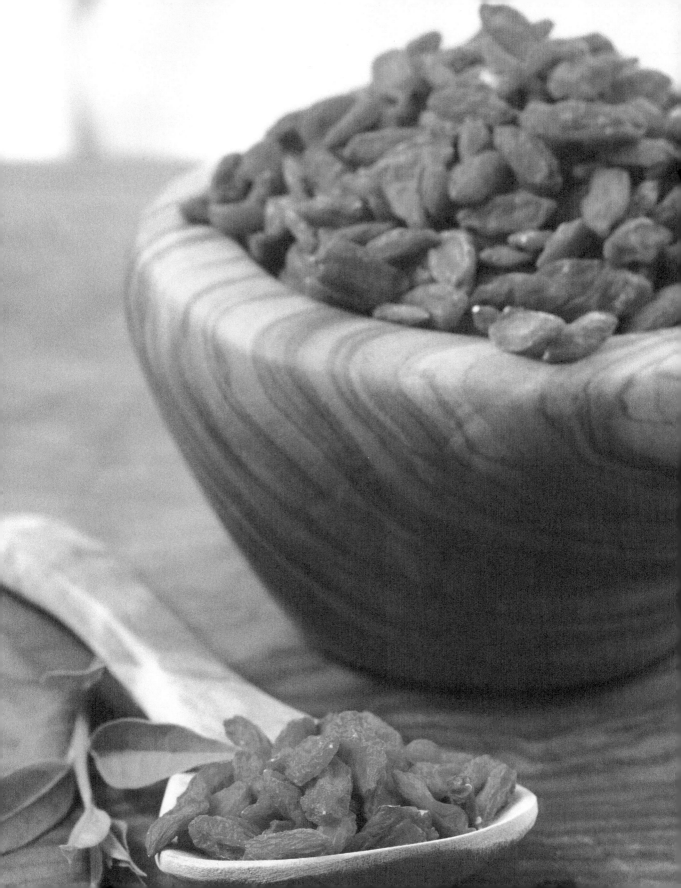

Go Green
The Superfood Organic Green Powder

Go Green is an alkalising organic Super Green blend which includes Wheat Grass, Barley Grass, Lucuma, Spearmint and Banana powder.

It has been formulated to assist the body with its natural detoxification processes and will also boost immunity and help with energy production.

It contains dietary fibre and is rich in B vitamins, Vitamins C and E, iron and zinc.

This cleansing Superfood blend will also assist with satiety, will help to control cravings and will help to regulate digestive function.

Go Green can be taken once or twice daily in a little water or can be added to one of your daily juices or smoothies.

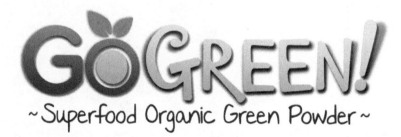

Go Boost is available from **www.thesuperfoodist.com**

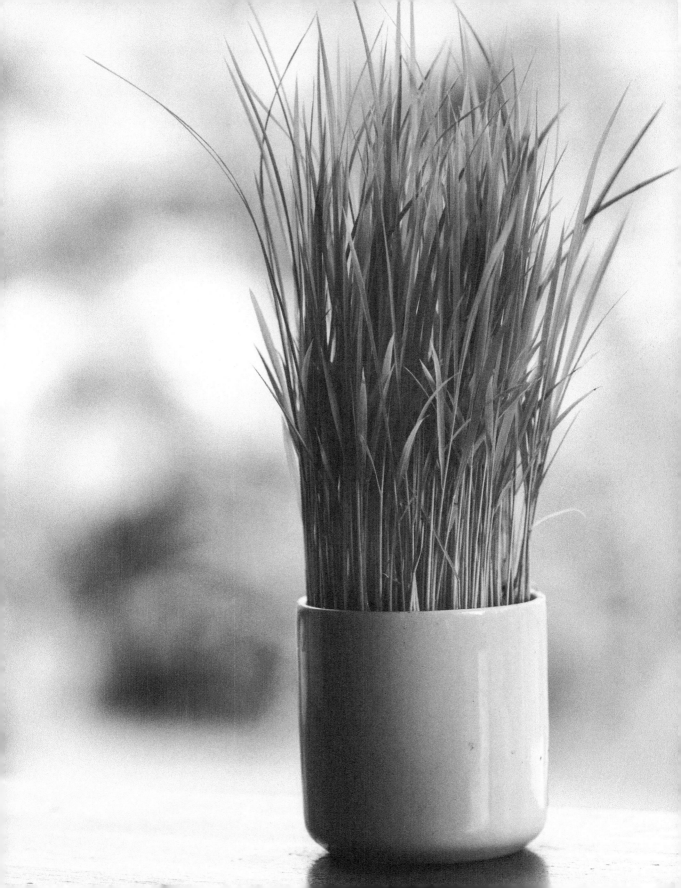

Fushi

Rick is the Nutritional Formulator for Fushi's supplement range in London.

His Nutraceutical formulas have won many awards and include Beauty Totale, The Best Super Food Berry Blend, Cellufirm, Dietone, Cardio Tatale and The Best Fibre Food Blend.

These nutraceuticals can be used in conjunction with The Anti Ageing Food and Fitness Plan to address any specific health areas that may need some extra support.

He is also the co formulator of Believe Beauty Breakfast Cereal, which contains seventeen important vitamins, minerals and superfoods to promote healthy hair, skin and nails.

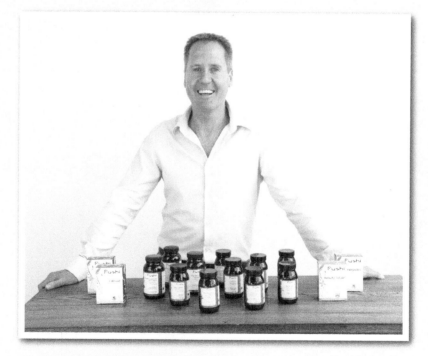

www.thesuperfoodist.com

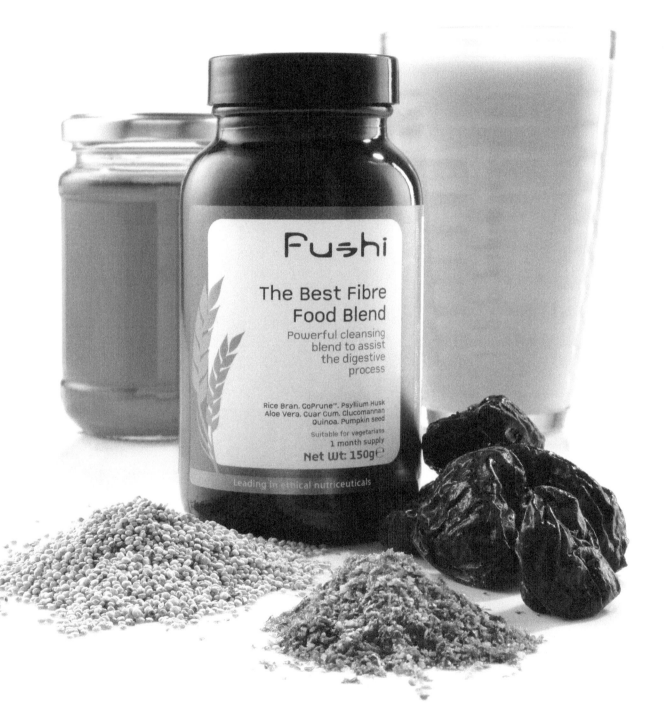

Fushi

The Best Fibre Food Blend

Powerful cleansing
blend to assist
the digestive
process

Rice Bran. GoPrune™. Psyllium Husk
Aloe Vera. Guar Gum. Glucomannan
Quinoa. Pumpkin seed

Suitable for vegetarians
1 month supply
Net Wt: 150g℮

Leading in ethical nutriceuticals

Sunwarrior Plant Based Protein

Sunwarrior Plant Based Protein comes in Warrior Blend – a mix of cold extracted Hemp, Pea and Cranberry with additional nutritional co factors. Alternatively, there is the Classic Protein which is derived from sprouted Organic Brown Rice.
Both varieties are rich in amino acids and are available in Vanilla, Chocolate or Natural flavour.

Sunwarrior Protein is easily digestible and is full of vitamins, minerals, amino acids and phytonutrients.
These nutrients nourish the body at a cellular level and assist in fighting the free radicals that are responsible for so much of the ageing process.

Sunwarrior can be taken as a meal or snack replacement to help with weight management goals. It can also be taken as part of a fitness programme - pre or post workout - to assist with lean muscle gain and toning.

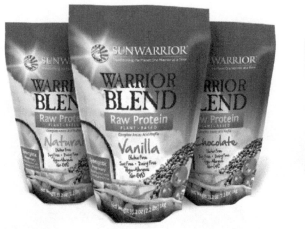
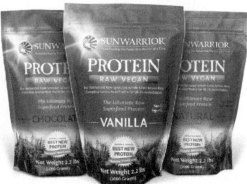

www.thesuperfoodist.com

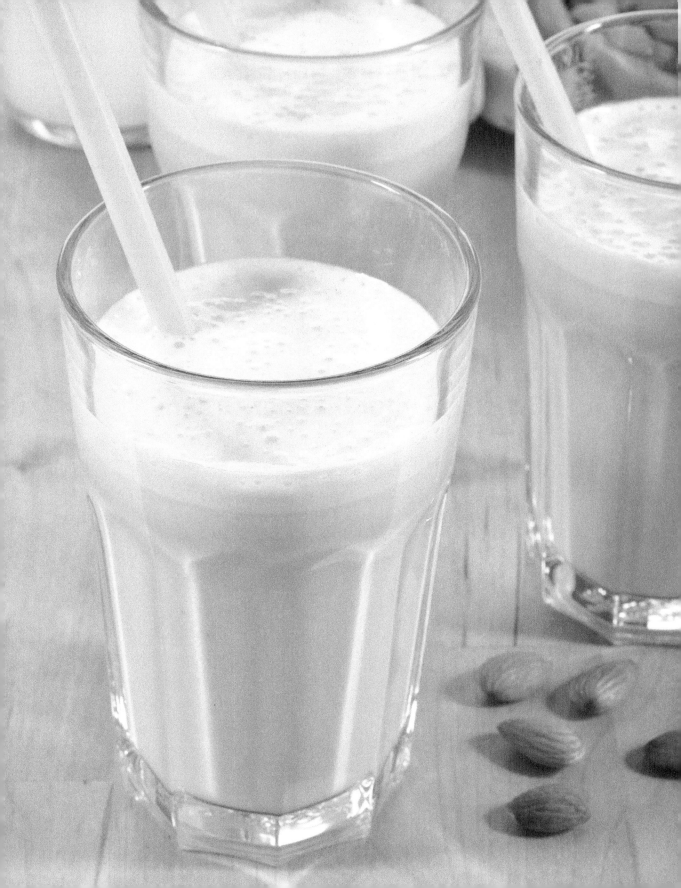

Synergy Natural Spirulina

Spirulina was originally discovered growing naturally on unpolluted alkaline lakes in Central Africa and Mexico where it was integrated into the diet of the mighty Aztec empire.

Today Spirulina (*Arthrospira platensis*) is grown in large cultivated ponds in various tropical high sunshine areas around the world.

The best producers use certified organic, plant derived food, and ecologically sensitive practices for growing Spirulina.

Synergy Natural Spirulina is produced by the world's first and largest producer of Spirulina.

Extensive research and development over twenty years has resulted in a Spirulina with the highest levels of all nutrients.

It is grown ecologically without pesticides or herbicides and carefully dried in a few seconds preserving full nutritional value without any chemical additives.

Synergy Natural Super Greens

Synergy Natural Super Greens is a synergistic blend of Nature's most nutrient dense green superfoods, Spirulina, Chlorella, Barley Grass and Wheat Grass.

Synergy Natural Super Greens provides a wide spectrum of highly bio-available whole food nutrients, balanced by nature, that are absorbed more effectively than those found in synthetic formulations.

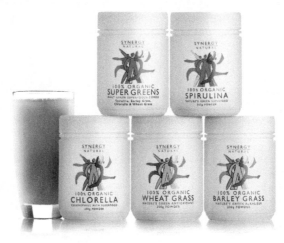

www.thesuperfoodist.com

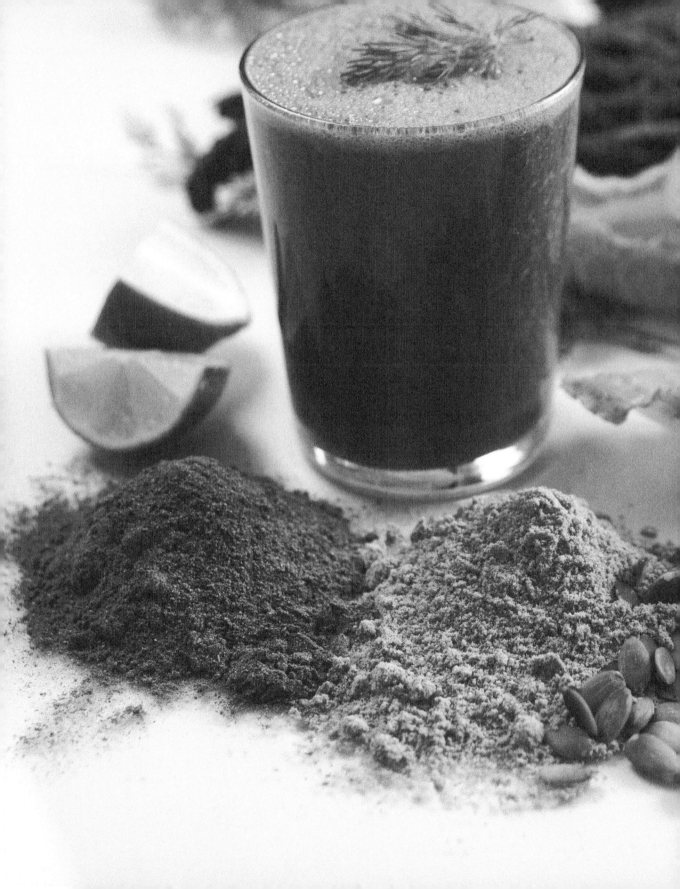

AminoGenesis
Fighting Glycation

If you eat lots of sugar and refined carbohydrates such as white rice, bread and pasta, levels of blood sugar in the body become high and remain so.

As a result, sugar molecules permanently bond to proteins, including the collagen in the skin – a process known as glycation.

This produces a chemical reaction in the skin that makes its surface more stiff and inflexible, leading to premature ageing making skin tougher and more wrinkled.

Glycation is damage to the skin from the inside due to the consumption of excess sugar.
It results in the three signs of ageing that we don't want – wrinkles, lines and discolouration. It can even lead to your skin becoming saggier as both collagen and elastin are damaged and become misshapen.

A.G.E. Control by AminoGenesis has been shown to help stop the glycation process and also help reverse the damage to important skin proteins like collagen and elastin.

www.thesuperfoodist.com

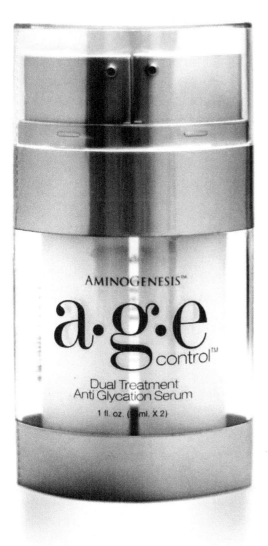
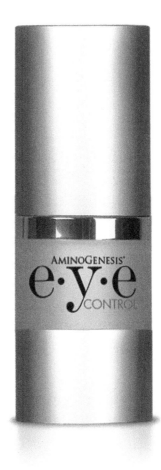

Superfood Combinations

The term 'superfood' has become a popular way to refer to nutritional powerhouses that have been shown to provide us with an array of antioxidants, phytonutrients, vitamins, minerals, enzymes and amino acids. Whether you want more energy, better immunity, weight management or to assist with digestive function, taking a superfood may help as they can provide concentrated levels of nutrients in freeze-dried powdered form and help supplement your diet with nutrients and you can achieve even better results if you combine two or three of them together.

Here are five of the best superfood combinations I've discovered:

Energy
Spirulina, Maca and Wheat Grass

Chlorophyll rich Spirulina and wheatgrass contain high levels of magnesium which boosts energy production at a cellular level. When combined with the amino acid dense South American superfood Maca these three make a great pre-exercise option – a nutrient dense natural energy drink that's caffeine and sugar free. This blend will also help promote lean muscle mass after exercise which assists in fat metabolism and toning.

Weight Loss
Chia Seeds and Spirulina

Add a teaspoon of Chia seeds and one of Spirulina to a smoothie in the morning to help kick start your metabolism. They are high in Omega 3 fatty acids so they will help with healthy hair, skin and nails and cognition and they also help balance blood sugar which means they could help keep cravings at bay. They swell slightly when added to liquid – this makes you feel fuller. The addition of spirulina to any smoothie also assists with satiety. Supergreen Spirulina also promotes healthy digestion which in turn assists with optimum fat metabolism.

Anti-Ageing
Cacao, Blueberry and Raspberries

This trio contains bioflavonoids, anthocyanidins and resveratrol – superbly powerful antioxidants that may help the body protect and repair itself. These produce positive benefits in terms of protecting the length of your 'telomeres' – little tips at the ends of your chromosomes that scientists have found shorten as the body ages. Longer healthy telomeres mean a longer healthy life. The coloured pigments in the berries are what provide the antioxidant content and combine wonderfully with the cardioprotective nature of the cacao – the raw cacao protects against toxins and can repair damage caused by free radicals.

Digestion
Barley Grass, Aloe Vera and Turmeric

To help reduce bloating and digestive problems add a half a teaspoon of barleygrass and half a teaspoon of turmeric powder to a smoothie or juice and drink once or twice a day – add 5mls of antiviral, antimicrobial and antibacterial aloe vera juice to help soothe an upset tummy and to reduce flatulence. They also have prebiotic qualities that will encourage the growth of gut friendly probiotics. Meanwhile, turmeric contains a substance called curcumin which has been shown to work as a powerful anti-inflammatory.

Detox
Chlorophyll, Wheat Grass, Barley Grass and Spirulina

Clean and alkalise the system with these four supergreens. You only need to add a quarter of a teaspoon of each to water or fresh juice to create a Ph-balancing nutritional cocktail that will help to alkalise your system – great if you've been overdoing it on coffee, sweets and meat or if you're under extreme stress as all these make your body overly acidic. The key to these superfoods is their deep green colour; the pigments come from enzymes in the foods that help to create optimum digestion and elimination.

Keep Your Body Young

Talk to any anti-ageing scientist right now and they'll mention telomeres. The longer yours are the better – and the slower you will age. Telomeres are like protective bookends on the end of our chromosomes. Long healthy ones appear to be the key to protecting against age related illnesses and some would say they could be the key to slowing the ageing process itself.

You might have heard of the antioxidant resveratrol - rich quanitities are in dark green and purple foods such as blueberries and grapes (and red wine). Resveratrol has been shown to both protect and lengthen telomeres.

I'm an advocate of a good glass of red every night with dinner but to get sufficient therapeutic amounts of resveratrol you'd have to drink hundreds of bottles which kind of negates the health benefits of the red wine! You can purchase resveratrol as a supplement but antioxidants are best taken from foods rather than in pills so if you're opting for a supplement, check it's food derived not synthetically produced.

There are other foods and nutrients that may assist in protecting telomeres and in the activation of telomerase. Telomerase is an enzyme that keeps your telomeres in good shape and by having healthy lengthy telomeres, you will hopefully be protected from many age-related illnesses.

These foods not only protect telomeres but ongoing research is indicating that these nutrients that help lengthen telomeres also give you more energy and boost your immune system in general.

Here are my top tasty telomere-boosting nutrients, which I advise you to try to incorporate into your diet on a daily basis:

1. Antioxidants

Studies have shown that longer telomeres are associated with high antioxidant and polyphenol intake so think berries, wheatgrass, barleygrass, Chlorella, turmeric, hemp protein, astaxanthin, co-enzyme Q10, green tea or organic cacao.

2. Vitamin D Rich Foods

Foods that are high in Vitamin D are also telomere protectors – these include fish, tofu, eggs, oysters, mushrooms - and caviar if you're feeling extravagant.

3. Folate

Lentils and spinach are perfect as they are high in folate, which promotes telomere health. Spinach makes a great addition to any juice or smoothie and lentils are a great source of protein and fibre to add to any soup.

4. Magnesium

This mineral is believed to influence telomere length by helping with the integrity and repair of DNA so keep up your intake of dark leafy greens, nuts, seeds, avocados, bananas and figs.

Keeping stress at bay will also help with telomere length and plays a key part in slowing down ageing. Life's too short not to indulge from time to time so when you've enjoyed that glass of red wine with dinner why not have a piece of dark organic chocolate for dessert as that delicious, dark organic chocolate is also rich in magnesium.

Beat the Bloat
My 12 essential tips to beat the bloat

1. Take probiotics

These aid digestion, mood and boost immunity too – but most importantly they reduce gas-producing bacterial imbalances thereby helping to keep the tummy flat.

2. Relax

Stress causes a build up of cortisol and adrenaline which can over stimulate your digestive system leading to flatulence and bloating – think Yoga or even a candle lit bath with some magnesium rich Epsom salts or relaxing essential oils.

3. Do core exercises

Strong abs inhibit gas from pushing outwards resulting in less tummy distension.

4. Decrease your dairy intake

As one of the main symptoms of lactose intolerance is bloating, decreasing your intake of diary products is a good first step. There's lots of dairy alternatives like gut soothing rice milk or coconut yogurt that can be included into your bloat busting diet. You could decrease wheat too as wheat products can be quite challenging to the digestive system for many individuals. Stay clear of dairy products to prevent bloating

5. Eat bananas, kiwis and strawberries

These are high in potassium which acts as a diuretic and increases the amount of salt in your urine – that's good news as excess salt can cause water retention in the small intestine. Kiwis and strawberries are the way the forward.

6. Stop talking when eating

Tough we know, swallowing air causes bloating.

7. Skip the gum

Chewing gum that contains xylitol, sorbitol or mannitol can increase the production of gas in the digestive tract.

8. Try the herb Vitex Berry (Chaste Tree)

It can help decrease hormonal bloating. It's best taken as a tincture or tea with meals. This herb has been used traditionally to treat irregular menstruation.

9. Eat fewer bloating foods

Cut down on consumption of beans, onions, broccoli, cabbage, sprouts and cauliflower as these are known gas-producing foods. Instead, apples, pears and melon, which are pectin rich – this is a calming substitute that will keep your fibre levels up. Take probiotics and vegetable digestive enzymes to help balance the gut whilst you reduce these foods then you can increase them slowly. Foods such as beans will increase bloating.

10. Take vegetable digestive enzymes

These help balance the stomach and relieve any symptoms, including heartburn and indigestion.

11. Try Aloe Vera juice

This is my top gut soother – it detoxifies, it's anti microbial, anti bacterial and anti viral too. This plant reduces internal inflammation and as a bonus can help improve skin conditions like eczema and rosacea too.

12. Get checked for Coeliac disease

See your GP for a blood test if you suspect gluten may be behind your discomfort. If this proves negative, it may be worth having a food intolerance test. The York Test is a test you can do by mail that identifies foods you could be intolerant to, which may be causing your bloating, wind and cramping.

Natural Face Lift
Reduce Sugar and Glycation

Sugar has become nutritional public enemy number one. But quite aside from making you fat, evidence suggests it could also affect the skin.

When you eat lots of sugar and refined carbohydrates such as white rice, bread and pasta, levels of blood sugar in the body become high and remain so. As a result, sugar molecules permanently bond to proteins, including the collagen in the skin – a process known as glycation. This produces a chemical reaction in the skin that makes its surface more stiff and inflexible, leading to premature ageing making skin tougher and more wrinkled.

Glycation leads to wrinkles, lines, discolouration and even to saggier skin as collagen and elastin are compromised.

A study published in the Journal of the American College of Nutrition, in which researchers studied the diets of 453 adults living in different countries, found that those who consumed more fish, olive oil and legumes were less prone to wrinkles than those who ate more meat, butter, high fat dairy and sugar.

In particular, processed meat, soft drinks and pastries were associated with more skin wrinkling, while beans, green leafy vegetables, asparagus, nuts, olives, apples and pears were associated with less skin ageing.

Advanced glycation end products or (appropriate acronym of the century) AGEs not only cause protein fibres to become malformed they also contribute to connective tissue damage, chronic inflammation, heart disease and diabetes.

Intrigued by this information I spoke to Ron Cummings, CEO of AminoGenesis skin care, who told me that he believed that glycation was even more detrimental to skin health than is oxidation, which we've all been talking about for the last decade as skin's number one health enemy.

Diet and lifestyle choices can affect how quickly the effects of glycation can be seen on the skin so avoid a high glycaemic load diet that's high in sugar and refined carbohydrates, smoking, processed foods and meats, excess alcohol and foods that have been deep fried.

It's all about limiting excess sugar intake and reducing both oxidative stress and oxidisation. Try too to stay away from high-fructose corn syrup as studies have shown that this sweetener significantly increases the rate of glycation – it's in fizzy drinks and many processed sweets.

The good news is that it that once a protein has been glycated it can be repaired. You can use a serum that will fight glycation when applied topically: Age Control is one formula that helps break the chemical bond between the sugar molecule and the protein, which allows the protein to recover. This formula uses an extract from the mimosa plant due to its anti-glycation properties.

A Mediterranean Diet that focuses on fresh fruit and vegetables, whole grains and lean protein will help to reduce inflammation and provide high levels of the free radical fighting vitamin trio – A, C and E. The Anti Ageing Food and Fitness Plan is another option as this combination of nutrient rich foods and simple exercise routines will help fight the glycation process.

You should drink a cup or two of green tea each day as this is a powerful skin protector that stimulates collagen production, and consume more tomatoes as they are high in lycopene, which has an anti-glycation action.

You can increase dietary levels of the amino acid carnosine by consuming more fish, organic cheese and eggs. Carnosine has been shown to protect against the damaging effects of AGEs.

Other foods to consume to help tighten that saggy glycated skin include, avocados, mackerel, berries and garlic.

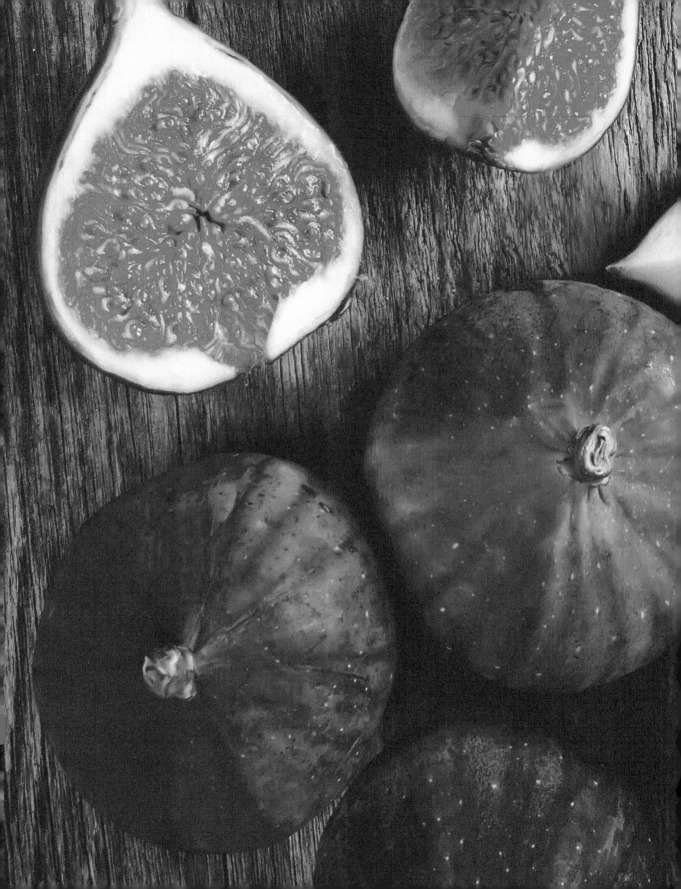

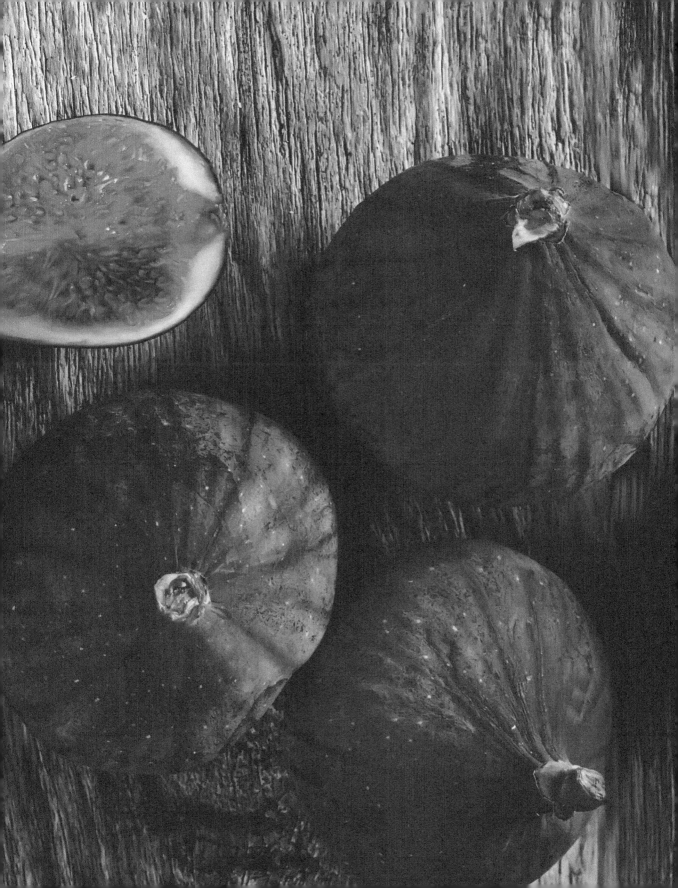

Energy Booster

- ~ Half an avocado
- ~ 2 Cups of spinach
- ~ 5 or 6 Cashews
- ~ 1 Small nectarine or plum
- ~ 1 teaspoon of linseeds
- ~ 6 or 7 Red or green grapes
- ~ 200 mls of coconut water

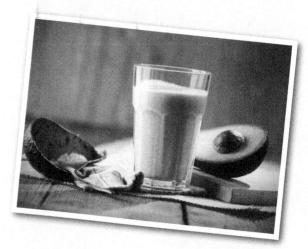

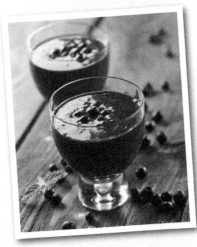

Spice Up

- ~ 1 Cup mixed berries
- ~ 1 Cup of mixed leafy greens
- ~ 1 Teaspoon of sunflower or pumpkin seeds
- ~ 7 or 8 Almonds
- ~ A pinch of chilli or cayenne if desired
  Turbocharge with a teaspoon of wheat grass powder
- ~ 200 mls of Unsweetened almond milk

Pre-Workout Berry Blast

- ~ 1 Cup strawberries
- ~ 1 Cup raspberries
- ~ 7 or 8 Almonds
- ~ 1 Teaspoon sunflower or pumpkin seeds
- ~ 1 Cup leafy greens
- ~ Spinach or kale
- ~ Half a small beetroot
- ~ 200 mls of coconut milk or water

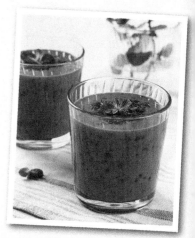

Raspberry Cacao Treat

~ 2 Cups raspberries

~ 1 Cup spinach

~ 2 Teaspoons cacao

~ 2 Teaspoons chia seeds

~ 1 Teaspoon sesame seeds

~ 1 Small beetroot

~ 200 mls of Water

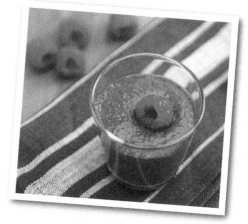

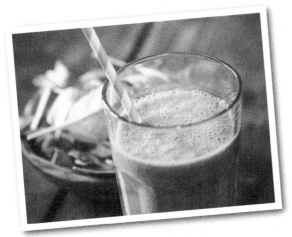

Green Dream

~ 1 Pear

~ 2 Celery stalks

~ 1 Inch slice of ginger

~ 2 Cups spinach or chard

~ 1/2 Avocado

~ 1 Teaspoon chia seeds

~ 200 mls Coconut water

Digestive Cleanse

~ 1 Pear

~ 1 Kiwi fruit

~ 2 Cups of spinach or lettuce

~ 200 mls Water

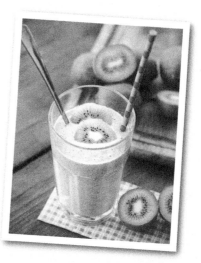

Ideal World TV

Rick is the Resident Health and Fitness Expert for Ideal World TV.
He appears regularly on both Vibrapower and Nutribullet Shows.

Ideal World TV have released Rick's 3 Vibrapower Fitness DVDs and
his Nutritional Blast Recipe Book.
His Nutraceutical formulations are also regularly featured on the
shows.

Details of Rick's appearances can be found on the Ideal World
website **www.idealworld.tv** or on the **Ideal World App**.

Websites and Social Media

Websites: www.thesuperfoodist.com *or* www.rickhay.co.uk

Facebook: Anti Ageing Food & Fitness

Twitter: @nutritionalphys

Instagram: rickhayuk *&* superfoodist

Blogs: wwww.healthista.com

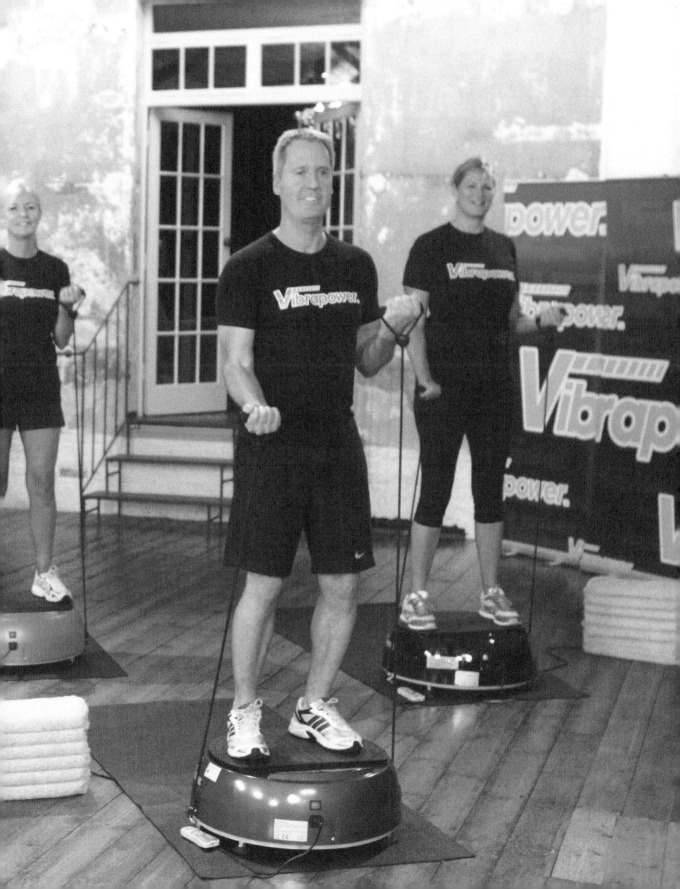

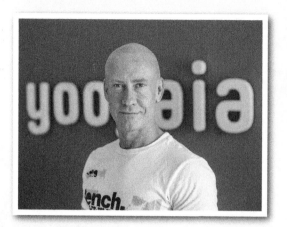

Ian Chapman
Anti Ageing Food & Fitness Plan Fitness Advisor

Ian Chapman created the fitness sections in the Anti Ageing Food & Fitness Plan.

He is a fully qualified, award winning Master Trainer, as well as a Yoga and Pilates teacher, with over 10 years experience in the Health and Fitness Industry.

Ian has worked internationally on a Luxury Cruise Liner, in small 1-to-1 studio spaces, in large commercial gyms and in corporate offices.

As well as writing his own fitness blog and shooting accompanying videos, Ian also guest presents fitness equipment on TV in Australia and in the UK.

Ian is currently the UK Manager of Yoogaia - the first online live yoga studio in the world that brings yoga, pilates, core and barre classes to your home in real-time.

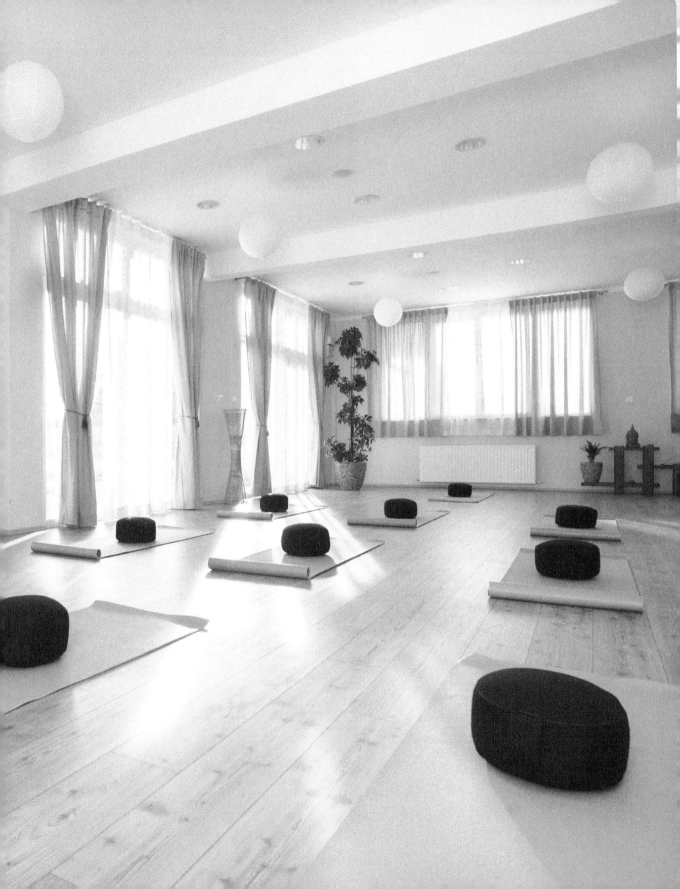

Lightning Source UK Ltd.
Milton Keynes UK
UKOW07f0612200616

276631UK00001B/4/P